WHY MOTHERS DIED AND HOW THEIR LIVES ARE SAVED

Why Mothers Died and How Their Lives Are Saved

The Story of Confidential Enquiries into Maternal Deaths

JAMES OWEN DRIFE
University of Leeds

GWYNETH LEWIS
University College London

JAMES NEILSON
University of Liverpool

MARIAN KNIGHT
National Perinatal Epidemiology Unit, Oxford

GRISELDA COOPER
University of Birmingham

ROCH CANTWELL
Perinatal Mental Health Network, NHS Scotland

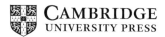
CAMBRIDGE
UNIVERSITY PRESS

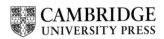

Shaftesbury Road, Cambridge CB2 8EA, United Kingdom

One Liberty Plaza, 20th Floor, New York, NY 10006, USA

477 Williamstown Road, Port Melbourne, VIC 3207, Australia

314–321, 3rd Floor, Plot 3, Splendor Forum, Jasola District Centre, New Delhi – 110025, India

103 Penang Road, #05–06/07, Visioncrest Commercial, Singapore 238467

Cambridge University Press is part of Cambridge University Press & Assessment, a department of the University of Cambridge.

We share the University's mission to contribute to society through the pursuit of education, learning and research at the highest international levels of excellence.

www.cambridge.org
Information on this title: www.cambridge.org/9781009218795

DOI: 10.1017/9781009218825

First published 2023

A catalogue record for this publication is available from the British Library

Library of Congress Cataloging-in-Publication data
Names: Drife, James O., 1947– author. | Lewis, Gwyneth, MFPHM, author. | Neilson, James P., author. | Knight, Marian, author. | Cooper, Griselda, author. | Cantwell, Roch, author.
Title: Why mothers died and how their lives are saved : the story of confidential enquiries into maternal deaths / James Owen Drife, Gwyneth Lewis, James P. Neilson, Marian Knight, Griselda Cooper, Roch Cantwell.
Description: Cambridge, United Kingdom ; New York, NY : Cambridge University Press, 2022. | Includes bibliographical references and index.
Identifiers: LCCN 2022033946 (print) | LCCN 2022033947 (ebook) | ISBN 9781009218832 (hardback) | ISBN 9781009218825 (epub)
Subjects: MESH: Maternal Death – history | Maternal Health Services – history | Maternal Health Services – legislation&jurisprudence |MaternalMortality – history | Maternal Health – history |History, 20th Century | History, 21st Century | United Kingdom | BISAC:MEDICAL / Gynecology & Obstetrics
Classification: LCC RG725 (print) | LCC RG725 (ebook) | NLM WQ 11 FA1 | DDC 618.7/9–dc23/eng/20221110
LC record available at https://lccn.loc.gov/2022033946
LC ebook record available at https://lccn.loc.gov/2022033947

ISBN   978-1-009-21883-2   Hardback
ISBN   978-1-009-21879-5   Paperback

CONTENTS

CONTRIBUTORS

Roch Cantwell MB BCh BAO FRCPsych
Consultant Perinatal Psychiatrist
Lead Clinician and Retired Consultant Psychiatrist, Perinatal Mental Health
Network Scotland, Edinburgh
Chapter 12: Psychiatric Illness

Griselda Cooper OBE FRCA FRCOG
Retired Senior Lecturer
University of Birmingham
Consultant Anaesthetist
Birmingham Women's Hospital
Chapter 11: Maternal Death due to Anaesthesia

James Drife MD FRCOG FRCPE FRCSE FFSRH FCOGSA
Emeritus Professor of Obstetrics and Gynaecology
University of Leeds
Chapter 1: Historical Background
Chapter 2: The First Steps
Chapter 3: How the Confidential Enquiries Evolved
Chapter 4: The Missing Chapter?
Chapter 5: How the Change Began
Chapter 8: The Story of Abortion
Chapter 9: Challenging Tradition
Chapter 10: Pregnancy and Illness

Marian Knight MA MBChB MPH DPhil FFPH FRCPE FRCOG
Professor of Maternal and Child Population Health
National Perinatal Epidemiology Unit
Oxford
Chapter 14: The Legacy in the United Kingdom

Gwyneth Lewis OBE DSc FRCOG FRCGP FFPHM FACOG
Retired Lead for International Women Health Research
University College London
Chapter 13: The Mothers Who Died
Chapter 15: International Maternal Health

Elliott Main MD
Medical Director
California Maternal Quality Care Collaborative
Clinical Professor of Obstetrics and Gynecology
Stanford University School of Medicine
Chapter 16: International Action

James Neilson MD FRCOG
Emeritus Professor of Obstetrics and Gynaecology
University of Liverpool
Chapter 6: Haemorrhage Then and Now
Chapter 7: Hypertension

Vakkaram Paily MBBS MD FRCOG
Past President
Kerala Federation of Obstetrics and Gynaecology
Senior Consultant and Head of Department of Obstetrics and Gynaecology
Rajagiri Hospital, Chunangamvely, Aluva, Kerala, India
Chapter 16: International Action

Robert Pattinson BSc MBChB MMed (O&G) MD FCOG(SA) FRCOG
Director, Maternal and Infant Health Care Strategies Unit
South Africa Medical Research Council
Emeritus Professor
Research Centre for Maternal, Fetal, Newborn & Child Health Care Strategies
Faculty of Health Sciences, University of Pretoria, Hatfield, South Africa
Chapter 16: International Action

FOREWORD

MAHMOUD FATHALLA

The story of 'Confidential Enquiries into Maternal Deaths' (CEMDs) had to be told and has to be heard, not only as a success record of a past that should not be forgotten, but as an inspiration for present and future action. As Winston Churchill rightly said, the longer you can look back, the farther you can look forward. Professor James Drife, Professor Gwyneth Lewis and their colleagues are to be congratulated for compiling the lessons of this 70-year story and giving recognition to those who richly deserve it.

The CEMDs revealed the inconvenient truth that mothers were not dying because of conditions we could not prevent or treat. The enquiries were confidential, but the findings were widely publicised to shame society into action, and so they did. In many parts of our world today, mothers still risk giving up their lives in the noble task of giving us a new life, and the question of why did they die continues to beg for answers and for remedial actions to correct this grave injustice.

The lessons of the CEMDs will be an inspiration for present and future leaders who continue to carry the torch of women's right to safe motherhood. The story will also appeal to a much wider audience interested to know more about pioneers who stood up to their social responsibility, changed history and made a difference in women's healthcare.

Professor Mahmoud Fathalla, MD PhD Hon FRCOG
Department of Obstetrics and Gynaecology, Assiut University, Egypt
Past President, International Federation of Gynecology and Obstetrics (FIGO)
Former Chairman, WHO Global Advisory Committee on Health Research

FOREWORD

DONNA OCKENDEN

Recent tragedies have cruelly reminded us that pregnancy still carries risks to mothers and their babies. The work to reduce these risks began a century ago, when death in childbirth was far more common than it is today. Maternal mortality remained stubbornly high until the 1920s, when demands grew for action. This book describes what happened next and reveals parallels with the present day.

The first step was a series of reports examining women's deaths and calling for better training of midwives and doctors. They were written by an all-female team of public health doctors. Pressure from them and women's organisations pushed the government into establishing a national enquiry. It examined thousands of deaths and made far-reaching recommendations.

Another groundbreaking innovation was involving women in their own care. In 1930 the industrial town of Rochdale had the highest rate of maternal death in the country. This was halved in two years, mainly by health education. Women (and men) were found to be 'intensely keen to be told the truth ... in simple straightforward language'.

Those reports began a pattern which continues to this day. The system improved and gave the public the facts with unflinching honesty. The Ministry of Health feared a hostile response, but from the start the reports of the Confidential Enquiries were welcomed by the public and the professions. They were harrowing, but they were read and – importantly – acted upon.

What comes across throughout this book is a shared sense of purpose. Doctors, midwives, women, politicians, activists and scientists worked together to revolutionise the safety of childbirth. But, as well as celebrating the pioneers, the book provides a timely reminder that the work must continue. Women are still dying needlessly in the UK and across the globe. Recent sobering lessons from today's UK Enquiries are set out in the later chapters, along with groundbreaking work in South Africa, India and the USA, where confidential enquiries have the potential to save many more lives.

I recommend this unique book to everyone interested in the safety of maternity care. Written by a team of experts, it explains 'in simple straightforward language' as was pioneered in the 1930s how we got to where we are today and why constant vigilance is essential to keep the mothers and babies of today safe.

Donna Ockenden
Chair, The Maternity Reviews
Shrewsbury and Telford Hospital NHS Trust
Nottingham University Hospitals NHS Trust

INTRODUCTION
GWYNETH LEWIS & JAMES DRIFE

One of the most dramatic changes in the life of women in the twentieth century was the advent of safe childbirth. In 1928 pregnancy caused the deaths of 2,920 women in England and Wales. In 2018 the UK figure was 72. Reducing the nation's maternal mortality rate from 1 in 400 to 1 in 10,000 births was a remarkable achievement. This book explains how it was done.

People often assume that the change was a by-product of an overall improvement in public health. In fact it was due to direct action, initiated by public outrage at a death rate that had remained unchanged since Queen Victoria took the throne.

It started with Senior Medical Officer Janet Campbell, appointed when the Ministry of Health was set up in 1919. She began with a detailed investigation into why women died, as described in Chapter 2. The next step was to educate poorly trained doctors.

Change was boosted by the discovery of antibiotics. Chapter 5 summarises the long battle against childbed fever, finally won during the Second World War when the maternal death rate fell faster than at any time before or since.

After the war the pioneers could have rested on their laurels. Instead they set up Confidential Enquiries into Maternal Deaths (CEMDs), which became the world's longest-running professional self-audit and a shining example for healthcare workers across the globe. Chapter 3 describes how it developed, and Chapter 4 explains some of the problems hidden in its early appendices.

One by one the causes of maternal death were tackled. Each required a different approach, as enumerated in Chapters 5–9. By 1961 the leading cause was abortion, and Chapter 8 tells the story of the people whose campaigning led to the Abortion Act of 1967.

Their names, like the names of Dame Janet and many others, faded from history despite the far-reaching consequences of their work. Men and women changed history and then all but disappeared. This book restores their place in the story of women's healthcare.

In the 1990s the CEMDs first revealed the vast disparities in outcomes for mothers of different ethnic groups and social classes which are explored in

Chapter 13 and have persisted to this day. The importance of postnatal depression was slowly recognised, as studied in Chapter 12. The original CEMD closed in 2011, but its work continues under MBRRACE and has expanded, as examined in Chapter 14. Constant vigilance remains essential.

All the authors of this book had leading roles in the work of the CEMD. Why have we decided to tell its story? We have chosen to do so partly to honour the memory of our predecessors, whose work saved lives and deserves to be acknowledged by the public as well as by their colleagues.

But there are more practical reasons. We can learn from success. The CEMD was a partnership between politicians, civil servants and professionals – and the public. Its enquiries were confidential, but its findings were not, and it had a flair for publicising them.

Global maternal mortality is still far too high. Chapter 15 looks at the international influence of the CEMD. Countries have had mixed success in implementing such enquiries, and Chapter 16 features personal reflections from colleagues working on different continents. We hope our book and their comments will help politicians and professionals make a real difference in countries where women are still dying needlessly in pregnancy.

1   HISTORICAL BACKGROUND

When Confidential Enquiries into Maternal Deaths (CEMDs) began in England and Wales in 1950, childbirth in the UK was entering a new era. The National Health Service (NHS) was two years old. The still-new colleges of midwives and obstetricians had just become 'Royal'. The age-old curse of puerperal sepsis had been lifted. Public protests about high death rates in childbirth and infancy had ended. Maternal mortality had begun to fall and the professions and the government were united in their resolve to make pregnancy even safer.

The task would not be easy. It would need the co-operation of midwives, general practitioners (GPs), obstetricians, hospital services and public health officials, and a controversial Act of Parliament. Each piece of that complex jigsaw has its own history, tacitly understood when the CEMD began making its recommendations but largely forgotten today. Some of those histories are mentioned in later chapters, but the background stories of midwives, doctors and hospitals are summarised here. They help to explain the conditions in which the new CEMD had to operate, and they may also make surprising reading.

The midwives

The word 'midwife' sounds feminine but actually it is gender neutral. It comes from the Middle English 'mid' (with) and 'wyfe' (woman) and simply means the person who is 'with the woman' at childbirth. For centuries, however, men were excluded from labour and birth, and the term 'midwife' came to cover a broad spectrum of birth attendants from trained professionals to the local 'handywoman'. The extremes are exemplified by two historical figures, one real and one fictitious.

Mrs Nihel and Mrs Gamp

Elizabeth Nihel was a leading midwife in the eighteenth century. She trained at the Hotel Dieu in Paris (one of the few midwifery schools of the time) before setting up in practice in London in 1749 and writing her own textbooks. She objected strongly to the rise of the 'man midwife' and has been immortalised by her picturesque comments about them.

Sarah Gamp appeared in Charles Dickens' novel *Martin Chuzzlewit*, published in 1843. Sloppy, ignorant and fond of gin, she combined the roles of midwife and nurse, and 'went to a lying-in or a laying-out with equal zest and relish'. Based on a real person a female friend had described to Dickens, she became a popular nineteenth-century stereotype.

Dickens' caricature, however, contained more than a grain of truth. In 1871 Florence Nightingale wrote, in her book *Notes on Lying-in Hospitals*:

> *Although every woman would prefer a woman to attend upon her in her lying-in, and in diseases peculiar to her and her children, yet the woman does not exist, or hardly exists, to do it. Midwives are so ignorant that it is almost a term of contempt.*

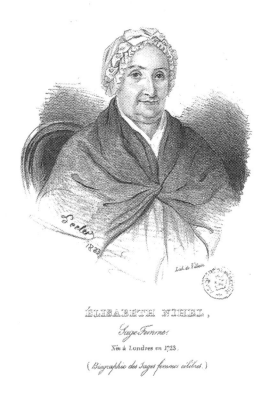

Figure 1.1 Mrs Elizabeth Nihel (1723–76)

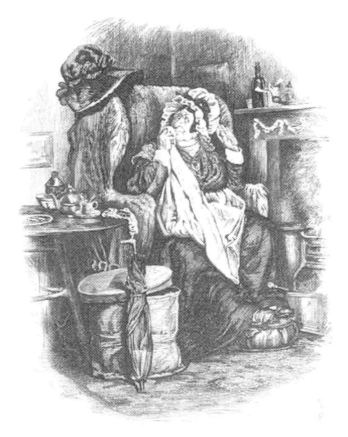

Figure 1.2 Sarah Gamp, as illustrated by Frederick Barnard

She had already turned nursing into a respected profession and she outlined the training required to do the same for midwifery. Her mission was taken up by others in the 1880s. The first step was to be a statutory register of midwives. The Medical Register had been established in 1858 to help people distinguish between professionals and quacks, and the Midwives Register would do the same. In 1890 a Midwifery Bill was presented to Parliament in the short-lived hope that it would pass with little debate.

The Midwives Act

The second reading was moved on 21 May 1890 by Liberal and Conservative Members of Parliament (MPs), who said their purpose was to ensure that the poor had access to the standards of midwifery that the rich already enjoyed. The bill was opposed, however, by a medically qualified MP who said he 'had received representations from medical men stating that the passage of this Bill would deprive them of much legitimate practice which they at present enjoyed'. It was talked out and 12 years of debate followed.

Doctors argued that there were no adequate facilities for midwife training. Some even formed the Committee to Oppose Midwives' Registration. Anti-female prejudice was rife at that time, but this argument was more about finance than feminism. Doctors and midwives were private practitioners competing for fees from people who could afford them.

When the Midwives Act was finally passed in 1902, the debate intensified. If a midwife called a GP to help with a difficult labour, did the husband have to pay both of them? And what about people who could not afford to pay at all? The Poor Law Act of 1834 had established Poor Law Guardians, and in 1908 the Medical Protection Society wrote to all 648 Boards of Guardians pointing out that they were obliged by law to pay a doctor summoned by a midwife. Some Boards did so, others refused, and many haggled.

But money was not the main problem. Training had to be expanded rapidly and facilities were limited indeed. Formal midwifery training had been established in London in 1872, when the London Obstetrical Society introduced a diploma specifically for midwives. This had been a controversial step. A leading obstetrician, Sir Francis Champneys, later recalled that, as the president of the Society, he had signed the diplomas personally and some doctors had threatened to refer him to the General Medical Council for doing so. Champneys was intent on raising the status of midwives and he became a driving force behind the Midwifery Act.

Zepherina Smith

Among the first to receive the Society's diploma was a nurse, Zepherina Veitch, who had already published *A Handbook for Nursing the Sick*. In 1881, encouraged by the activist Louisa Hubbard, she and six other midwifery diplomates formed the Matron's Aid Society to improve the training of midwives. They chose that name because the word 'midwife' was rarely used in polite society.

Soon the Society gained the confidence to rename itself the Midwives Institute and in 1890 Zepherina (by then Mrs Smith) became its president. She attended meetings of the committee which framed the Midwives Bill but did not live to see it become law. She died in 1894, aged 58, but the Institute continued and became the College of Midwives in 1941.

By 1902 schools of midwifery had been established outside London, including one in Liverpool, where formerly 'students were compelled to take out their course of practical midwifery in Dublin'. Ireland was well ahead of England

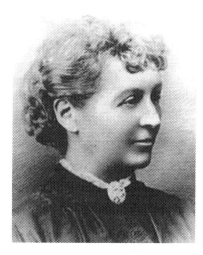

Figure 1.3 Zepherina Smith (1836–94)

and midwifery training had existed in Dublin since 1745, when the Rotunda Hospital was founded there.

The Central Midwives Board

The Midwives Act established the Central Midwives Board (CMB) to regulate the new profession. It included representatives from the two medical Royal Colleges, the Society of Apothecaries, nurses, laypeople and midwives. Champneys was its first chairman and was re-elected annually until his death in 1930 at the age of 82. According to an obstetrician colleague, William Fletcher Shaw, 'it was his administrative ability, patience, firmness, and tact which made possible the implementation of the Act'.

Balance and tact were indeed essential. Florence Nightingale had taken a gradual approach to the transformation of nursing by establishing a school in London and then sending her nurses to other cities. In complete contrast, the CMB appointed 'inspectors of midwifery' across the whole country simultaneously in 1905. As Shaw pointed out, this could have gone badly wrong. 'To have removed from the register all who failed to conform to modern standards before new ones had been trained would have created chaos: to have been too lenient and weak would have failed to bring home to the profession the necessity of improvement if they were to retain their registration.'

Thanks to Champneys, chaos was avoided. Shaw recalled that most of those who were reported to the CMB were 'admonished by the chairman, and dismissed with a caution, always with good effect'.

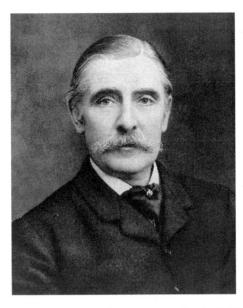

Figure 1.4 Sir Francis Champneys (1848–1930)

Gradually the length of midwifery training increased, standards were raised and better applicants were attracted. As midwifery became more autonomous the number of obstetricians on the Board reduced. In 1983 the CMB was replaced by the UK Central Council for Nursing Midwifery and Health Visiting, which in turn became the Nursing and Midwifery Council in 2002. By then midwifery was a graduate profession with (for better or worse) hardly any obstetric input into its degree courses.

The doctors

Obstetric teaching dates back to Hippocrates, but it almost disappeared in the Middle Ages when men were barred from childbirth and women were barred from universities. It re-emerged in Europe in the sixteenth century. Textbooks were printed in German and Latin, the surgeon Ambroise Paré founded a school for midwives in Paris, and accoucheurs (male midwives) appeared in France.

One of them was Peter Chamberlen, a Huguenot whose family fled to England in 1569. He became accoucheur to the Queen in 1616 and invented the obstetric forceps, which remained the Chamberlens' family secret for four generations. In the 1720s a great-grandson with no male heir divulged the design, and the use of forceps began to spread among the man-midwives who by then were becoming fashionable in England.

William Smellie

The most influential of these was William Smellie, a Scots doctor who moved to London in 1738 to learn midwifery and went to Paris for further training. When he returned he gave courses of his own. The standard fee for a two-year course of lectures was 20 guineas (about £4,000 today), and he advertised that 'The Men and Women are taught at different hours.'

Smellie improved the forceps and wrote rules for using them which still apply today. His *Treatise on the Theory and Practice of Midwifery*, published in 1752, included the advice never to criticise a midwife but to become her 'real friend'. Not all midwives reciprocated. Smellie lacked social graces and Mrs Nihel memorably called him 'a great horse God-mother of a he-midwife'. In 1759 he returned to the peace and quiet of his home town, Lanark, but his reputation as 'the master of British midwifery' lives on.

Lying-in hospitals

Another of the early man-midwives, Sir Richard Manningham, established London's first lying-in beds in 1739 in the house next door to his home in Jermyn Street. In 1745 a purpose-built lying-in hospital was founded in Dublin and later became the Rotunda. Its founder was Bartholomew Mosse, and, according to his biography, 'The wretchedness of the circumstances of many of the women that Mosse attended moved him deeply and he decided in the early 1740s to establish a charitable lying-in hospital.'

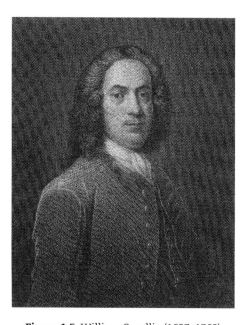

Figure 1.5 William Smellie (1697–1763)

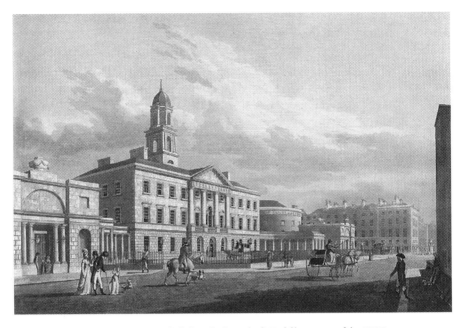

Figure 1.6 Rotunda lying-in hospital, Dublin, opened in 1757

London soon followed. The Middlesex Hospital added lying-in wards in 1747 and within five years there were five lying-in hospitals. They included the Bayswater Lying-in Hospital, which later became Queen Charlotte's and, like the Rotunda, offered midwifery training. As the Industrial Revolution progressed, other cities realised that their fetid slums were no place to have a baby. Lying-in hospitals were established in Newcastle, Manchester and Edinburgh, and later in Leeds, Liverpool and Sheffield.

The first medical schools

Until the eighteenth century Britain had no medical schools. Clinical teaching was available elsewhere in Europe or in one of London's two hospitals, St Bartholomew's and St Thomas', neither of which had a lying-in ward. Medicine in England was controlled by the Royal College of Physicians, which was founded in 1518 and did not regard midwifery as part of medicine. The surgeons had a trade guild that dated back to 1540 and would become a Royal College in 1800. They too eschewed midwifery, commenting that the only operation a man-midwife did was to cut the umbilical cord.

Britain's first medical school was founded in Edinburgh in 1726. Elsewhere in Scotland, Glasgow and Aberdeen followed in 1751 and 1786. In London, St

George's Hospital offered teaching from its foundation in 1733 and the London Hospital Medical College was founded in 1785. Edinburgh had a professor of midwifery from the start but London had no university until 1826, when University College was founded. In 1842 it appointed a Dublin-trained obstetrician as its first professor of midwifery.

Nineteenth-century innovation

During the nineteenth century the name 'man-midwife' was replaced by 'obstetrician', which comes from the Latin (*obstetrix* ('midwife')) and therefore has more gravitas. The century brought major innovations. Ether anaesthesia was discovered in 1846 by an American dentist, and chloroform anaesthesia was discovered in 1847 by the professor of midwifery in Edinburgh, James Young Simpson. The idea of pain relief in labour was briefly resisted on religious grounds, but when Queen Victoria asked John Snow for chloroform during her eighth labour in 1853 she set a trend that would continue into the twentieth century.

Joseph Lister pioneered aseptic surgery in the 1870s. It enabled abdominal operations and ushered in the specialty of gynaecology. The first successful hysterectomy in Europe had been performed in 1863 in Manchester, and in the 1870s a vogue developed for gynaecological procedures, many of them ill-advised by modern standards. Caesarean section remained rare, but isolated reports appeared from 1835 onwards. In 1894 a review of 160 caesarean sections in Britain and the USA reported mortality rates of 32–40%. *The Lancet* commented that it was 'still an operation attended with much danger'. This may have been because it was performed only as a last resort in the most difficult cases.

Undergraduate obstetrics

Between 1824 and 1834 seven new medical schools were established in quick succession across England but not all of them taught midwifery. Medicine was still dominated by the physicians and surgeons and was still an all-male profession. Women were excluded from the UK medical register until 1876 and from British universities until 1878. In such an atmosphere it is not surprising that the schools gave midwifery low priority. Later the honorary surgeon to Liverpool Maternity Hospital wrote: 'Obstetrics has always been the Cinderella of the Medical Faculty. It was considered a branch of the profession hardly respectable. The College of Physicians precluded practitioners of midwifery from their Fellowship; the College of Surgeons would not allow such a one to sit on its council until 1828.'

But the influence of obstetricians was growing. In 1824 they founded their own society, which became the Obstetrical Society of London in 1858, the year of the first Medical Act regulating medical education. In 1881 the Society's president, James Matthews Duncan (an Edinburgh alumnus), called for more curriculum time to be given to obstetrics and for the subject to have equal status with medicine and surgery.

Obstetrics finally became a statutory part of medical training in 1886, when a new Medical Act decreed: 'No person shall be registered under the Medical Acts who has not passed a qualifying examination in Medicine, Surgery, and Midwifery.' Ironically, four years later doctors were blocking the statutory training of midwives.

The birth of a specialty
By the 1870s the Obstetrical Society of London had about 600 members. It disapproved of the fad for gynaecological surgery and a breakaway group formed the British Gynaecological Society in 1884, but both became part of the Royal Society of Medicine in 1907. Regional societies were formed, such as the North of England Obstetrical and Gynaecological Society which was founded in 1889, and their proceedings were published in national journals.

In 1902 the specialty got its own journal. It had been suggested by Sir William Sinclair, an Aberdeen graduate who was a professor of obstetrics and gynaecology in Manchester. The first issue of the *Journal of Obstetrics and Gynaecology of the British Empire* devoted 30 pages to summaries of papers from abroad – 17 from France, 13 from Germany and 2 from the USA. This reflected the major sources of research in the specialty (and indeed in all medicine and surgery) at that time.

In 1911 William Blair-Bell of Liverpool formed the Gynaecological Visiting Society (GVS) with leading specialists from across Britain and Ireland. Blair-Bell had achieved national prominence because of his own research, but he is now remembered for founding the British College of Obstetricians and Gynaecologists in 1929. Among the other founding members were Sir Francis Champneys and William Fletcher Shaw.

Breaking away from the two established colleges was a bold step which needed a visionary leader. Blair-Bell was such a man: he became the College's first president and asked to be buried in the presidential robe he himself had designed. He died in 1936 and the College was granted its 'Royal' title in 1938, though it did not receive its charter until after the war.

In 1949 Dame Hilda Lloyd, Professor of Obstetrics and Gynaecology in Birmingham, became the Royal College of Obstetricians and Gynaecologists'(RCOG) first woman president. She had formed the Women's

Gynaecological Visiting Club in 1936 because women were excluded from the GVS and other national clubs. In 1949 Dame Hilda became the first woman to sit on the General Medical Council.

The RCOG quickly became an examining body like the other two colleges, with exacting standards in its membership examination. Candidates, however, had to rely on standard textbooks and local teaching. It was not until the 1990s that the RCOG began issuing its own guidelines on clinical practice.

Twentieth-century teaching

Although the 1886 Act had mandated midwifery teaching in medical schools, the subject struggled for curriculum time. In 1926 Sir Comyns Berkeley, a leading teacher and co-founder of the RCOG, inveighed against attitudes in London, where hospitals had far too few maternity beds for obstetric teaching, and he linked the neglect of midwifery teaching to the rate of maternal mortality, which was still scandalously high.

In 1930 the *Report of the Committee on Maternal Mortality and Morbidity* devoted a full chapter to medical education in obstetrics, and recommended improvements (see Chapter 2). In 1939 Sir John Fairbairn, another RCOG co-founder, called for a broader approach including preventive medicine. Commenting on the standards set by the CMB, he ended: 'Surely we teachers of medical students will not allow them to go into practice with a more restricted outlook than the midwives who will be their assistants.'

The General Practitioner Obstetrician

Medical school training was important because a newly qualified doctor could go directly into general practice. Before 1950 most births took place at home and maternity care was given by the midwife and GP. Who was 'assisting' whom is unclear. If pain relief was needed the midwife had to call the GP because the British Medical Association (BMA) had resisted calls to allow midwives to give any form of sedation.

Fairbairn pointed out that the GP saw his duty as relieving distress, usually by 'anaesthesia and a speedy and artificial end to labour'. This meant chloroform and forceps delivery, both of which carried risks, especially in the pre-antibiotic era. Postgraduate training in obstetrics or anaesthetics was not available and the GP obstetrician had to rely on his undergraduate teaching and then learn by experience.

When the NHS was set up in 1948 it proposed an 'obstetric list' of GPs with appropriate experience, who would receive extra remuneration. The BMA reluctantly agreed but then changed its mind. Throughout the 1950s its members repeatedly voted to abolish the list, arguing that all doctors learned enough at medical school to qualify for inclusion. Early signs of pregnancy complications continued to be missed, with fatal results.

The hospitals

St Bartholomew's and St Thomas' Hospitals were founded in the twelfth century, and London gained another hospital, Guy's, in 1721. The first general hospitals outside London were established in Bristol and York in 1735 and 1740, respectively, and over the next 50 years the expanding cities of the north of England did the same. Some of the cities also had lying-in hospitals. In the nineteenth century the term 'lying in' became obsolete and was replaced by 'maternity'.

Maternity hospitals

Between 1834 and 1842 maternity hospitals were established in Glasgow, Liverpool and Birmingham. In 1846 Edinburgh Lying-in Hospital changed its name to Edinburgh Royal Maternity Hospital. In 1865 Bristol Maternity Hospital was founded as The Temporary Home for Young Girls Who Have Gone Astray (later shortened to The Temporary Home). By 1875 maternity hospitals had been established in Sheffield, Aberdeen and Nottingham. Like the general hospitals, these were charitable institutions.

Maternity hospitals were bedevilled by outbreaks of puerperal fever (see Chapter 5), but infection was a problem in general hospitals too. Sir James Young Simpson coined the term 'hospitalism' for the complications that increased institutional mortality rates after amputations. Because sepsis was such a scourge it was suggested that all maternity hospitals should be closed down, but women were willing to take the risk and the hospitals expanded. In 1869 Glasgow Maternity Hospital reported that its births 'exceeded 1000 annually'.

Workhouse infirmaries

The poorest of the poor gave birth in workhouses, which had their origins in the fourteenth century. The Poor Law Act of 1834 entitled inmates to free medical care. Workhouses had a medical officer and, after another Act in 1867, they employed trained nurses. Many built their own infirmaries. In 1913 workhouses became 'Poor Law Institutions' and in 1929 the Boards of Guardians were abolished. The system ended with the National Assistance Act of 1948, but buildings repurposed as hospitals remained and, for the local people, so did the stigma.

A typical example was Leeds Workhouse, which opened in 1861. It added a block with lying-in beds to its infirmary in 1904. About 70 babies were born each year and the birth certificates carried a fictitious address. In 1925 the infirmary was renamed St James' Hospital. In 1934 it had 941 births but no resident obstetrician. In 1939 the government decided that the old Poor Law Infirmaries should have permanent medical staff but St James' did not get its own consultant obstetrician until 1953. He also covered one of the city's many maternity homes.

Maternity homes

Municipal maternity homes had been suggested in 1907 by Sir William Sinclair of Manchester, who had been a strong supporter of the Midwifery Act. In 1902, the year of the Act (and his new journal), the overwhelming majority of births were at home. Sinclair saw a need for maternity homes to which midwives' cases could be admitted if complications arose.

In 1919 the new Ministry of Health replaced the Local Government Board, and Janet Campbell (later Dame Janet) was appointed as the senior medical officer in charge of maternity and child welfare (see Chapter 2). By 1921 the Ministry had recognised 60–70 maternity homes in England and Wales and more were planned. Britain's maternal mortality rate was still high and Dame Janet believed that most maternal deaths could be prevented 'if proper facilities and reasonable skill were to hand'. She wanted maternity homes of 10–20 beds for 'normal and slightly abnormal cases' with good links to the local hospital, midwives and GPs.

She assumed these maternity homes would be well run, but the reality fell far short. In 1923 Beckwith Whitehouse (later Sir Beckwith), a Birmingham obstetrician and CMB examiner, drew attention to the poor standards in 'the types of maternity home which are springing up like mushrooms throughout the country, especially in the poorer areas of the large cities ... the small dirty house presided over by a woman frequently covered by the diploma of the CMB but without the experience needed to equip and manage a maternity home'.

In 1926 Parliament introduced registration making maternity homes liable to inspection by the supervising authorities established under an earlier Midwives Act. Complaints continued, however, particularly over the critically important issue of infection control. This is discussed in Chapter 5.

Another major issue was haemorrhage, which can occur suddenly at home or in a maternity home and needs immediate treatment. In 1929 Professor Farquhar Murray of Newcastle suggested that rather than rushing a shocked woman to hospital, a specialist and nurse should be rushed to the patient. The development of the 'obstetric flying squad' and its eventual demise are discussed in Chapter 6.

Summary

The eighteenth century gave Britain man-midwives, medical schools and hospitals. In the nineteenth century the medical profession became organised, anaesthesia was discovered, the germ theory of infection was proved and the specialty of obstetrics and gynaecology was born. In the twentieth century midwifery was transformed from a craft into a profession, the Ministry of Health was established and maternity homes were created.

Throughout all this, however, a woman's risk of dying in childbirth never changed. Maternal mortality in 1930 was as high as it had been in 1730. What did change was the public mood. Someone had to do something, and that is the subject of the next chapter in this story.

2 THE FIRST STEPS: 1900–1939

England has been recording the national rates of birth and death for a long time. Civil registration was introduced in 1837, replacing the parish registers which had kept records of christenings, burials and weddings since the reign of King Henry VIII. Under the new system the health of the whole nation, including religious nonconformists, could be monitored. From the 1840s onwards rates of maternal mortality (death of a woman during or just after pregnancy) and infant mortality (death before one year of age) were calculated and published. Both were tragically high and remained so until the 1900s.

During the nineteenth century Britain's expanding cities got clean water and built new sewage systems. Medical officers of health were appointed across the country. Workers' conditions were improved and child labour was ended. Nevertheless, despite all these public health measures, infant mortality scarcely changed, and it was infant death rather than maternal death that led to the first protests.

Infant mortality

In 1907 the National Association for the Prevention of Infant Mortality was formed. It grew in size and influence and in 1913 *The Lancet* reported a large attendance, including overseas representatives, at its meeting in Caxton Hall, Westminster. Co-chaired by a radical Member of Parliament (MP) and a marchioness, the meeting spanned the political and social divide. The MP, John Elliot Burns, was the sixteenth child in a family who had lived in a basement in Battersea after their father deserted them. The marchioness was the wife of Lord Aberdeen, former Viceroy of Ireland and ex-Governor General of Canada.

Both were concerned about the problems of the working class, particularly in the north of England. In Burnley the infant mortality rate was a staggering 171 per 1,000. In Battersea it was 83 and, as Burns pointed out, among doctors' babies it was 40. In towns and cities bottlefeeding was common but the milk was often contaminated, and Lady Aberdeen had long campaigned about this. Resolutions passed at the meeting included calls for the registration of stillbirths and for maternity benefits to be paid directly to mothers.

The first official enquiries

Already the government had begun to take action. Health at that time was the responsibility of the Local Government Board and in 1908 Dr Arthur Newsholme (a Yorkshireman) was appointed as its Medical Officer. In his first report he pointed out that one-fifth of all deaths in England were of infants in their first year of life. He swiftly introduced a system of enquiries into infant and child mortality in each of the nation's 54 administrative counties.

These enquiries confirmed that the main problem was in towns and cities. Rural and urban areas had the same rate of infant mortality in the first month of life but, between 6 and 12 months of age, the urban rate was 67% higher than the rural. Levels of poverty were similar in both areas but its effects were deadlier in towns. *The Lancet* commented that the main causes were over-crowding, bad housing and ignorance.

Campaigners believed that looking after a baby was not instinctive but a skill that had to be learned. In rural villages new mothers had the help of other women but city slums offered no such support system. Local authorities were pressed to establish classes in mothercraft – a word that had only just entered the language.

Motherhood and war

Infant mortality soon began to fall and in 1913 the Department published more detailed results of its enquiries – still without mentioning maternal mortality. Then the Great War brought new concerns. The British Army was losing hundreds of thousands of men in France and more babies were needed to replace them. The birth rate, however, had been falling since 1880, when accurate statistics were first published. *The Lancet* wrote about fears that 'the total number of the population would enter upon the downward path that leads to national extermination'.

In 1915 Dr Newsholme's report referred to 'the deplorable reduction in the fertility of English mothers'. *The Lancet*, under the title 'Motherhood, Infancy, and the War', called for efforts to solve the problem 'by preventing unnecessary wastage of infant life rather than by attempts at increasing the supply'. Realisation dawned that keeping mothers alive could also boost the war effort.

The first Maternal Mortality Enquiries

Dr Newsholme issued a supplementary report, *Maternal Mortality in Connection with Childbearing and Its Relation to Infant Mortality*. The maternal death rate was on average 4 per 1,000, or 1 in 250 births, and the report showed that 'infant mortality when mapped out for the whole country runs a course almost parallel with that of the death-rate among lying-in mothers'. On 20 November 1915 *The Lancet* noted that 'the subject of maternal mortality is now exciting daily increasing interest throughout the country'.

The leading cause of maternal death was puerperal infection, which had been compulsorily notifiable since 1899. Rates were similar across the country but the enquiries found that death from other causes was 'much higher in the provinces than in London, very probably because of the much greater accessibility there of skilled assistance in labour'. For example, in the northern textile towns of Rochdale and Dewsbury the maternal mortality rates were 8.5 and 7.2 per 1,000 births, respectively, compared with 3 per 1,000 in London.

At the end of the Report one of the Board's medical officers, Janet Lane-Claypon, discussed the impact of the maternity grant (introduced by the 1911 National Insurance Act) on midwives' fees and calls for medical assistance. Her colleague Isabella Cameron reported that, in lying-in hospitals, maternal mortality was 3 per 1,000, but, in charitable institutions providing midwifery care for home births, it was 1 per 1,000 or even lower.

The Lancet summarised the findings in detail and concluded: 'There can be no reasonable doubt that the quality and availability of skilled assistance before, during, and after labour are the most important factors in determining the serious differences in child-birth mortality.' But how was such skilled assistance to be provided?

Sir George Newman

By 1917 the government was planning post-war reconstruction. In 1919 the Local Government Board was replaced by a new national body, the Ministry of Health. Sir Arthur Newsholme retired and Sir George Newman, a Quaker and an Edinburgh medical graduate, was appointed as Britain's first Chief Medical Officer (see Figure 2.1). During his 16-year term of office maternal mortality became a top priority.

Newman was by nature a reformer. As the Medical Officer of Health in the London borough of Finsbury he had opened a milk depot which supplied not only clean milk but also education on hygiene. As medical officer to the Board of Education he had established a school medical service despite opposition

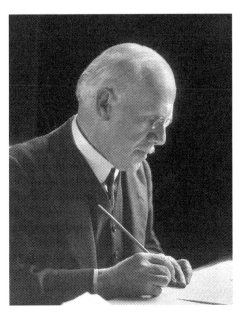

Figure 2.1 Sir George Newman (1870–1948)

from doctors in private practice. He had worked with the socialist Beatrice
Webb on a state medical service, which she proposed in a minority report of
the 1909 Royal Commission on the Poor Laws. The National Insurance Act of
1911 had fallen far short of this but was the first step on the road to the
National Health Service (NHS).

During the First World War Newman (by then Sir George) supervised the
health of munitions workers and established the Friends Ambulance Unit,
which allowed Quakers to serve as non-combatants on the front line. His crucial
contribution to the fight against maternal mortality came in 1919. When the
Ministry of Health was established he appointed Janet Campbell (later Dame
Janet) as the senior medical officer in charge of the Maternal and Child Welfare
Division, 'assisted by a staff of women doctors, nurses and midwives'.

Dame Janet Campbell

Janet Campbell, daughter of a Brighton bank manager, graduated MB
(Bachelor of Medicine) in 1901 from the London School of Medicine for
Women (see Figure 2.2). It had been founded by Sophia Jex-Blake, Elizabeth
Garrett Anderson and others and was the first school in Britain to train women
as doctors. Campbell went on from there to graduate, remarkably, as both MD
and MS (Doctor of Medicine and Master of Surgery). She worked at the Royal

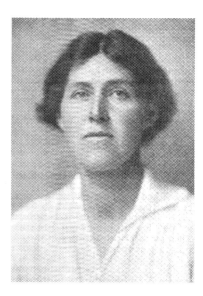

Figure 2.2 Dame Janet Campbell (1877–1954)

Free Hospital and in 1907 was appointed as the Board of Education's first woman medical officer. She was a founder member of the Medical Women's Federation and in 1924 she was made a Dame.

Dame Janet had a huge effect on women's health services in Britain and abroad, beginning with the series of reports she wrote at the Ministry of Health. Her 1923 report on medical students called for more maternity beds to be available for teaching and for 'the department of obstetrics and gynaecology to be a single whole and not divided'. This was ahead of its time: the *British Medical Journal* (BMJ) commented that 'an experiment in this direction made in Edinburgh was abandoned at the first opportunity'.

She then reported on midwives, suggesting that the training period 'for unqualified women should be extended from six months to twelve, and for trained nurses from four months to six'. Despite the Midwives Act of 1902, unqualified women were still attending maternity patients. Dame Janet suggested a midwifery teachers' certificate, which would at least ensure that the midwifery teachers had themselves practised as midwives.

The 1924 Report

Her most influential report, published in 1924, was *Maternal Mortality*. It was 112 pages long and attracted much attention. *The Lancet* published a summary followed by an editorial congratulating Dr Campbell on 'this valuable and painstaking report, a document which should be in the hands of all interested in the wellbeing of women and children, and which for this reason has been issued at the modest price of one shilling'.

The report highlighted the facts that maternal mortality had not changed since the nineteenth century and that the leading causes were sepsis, toxaemia and haemorrhage. *The Lancet* quoted evidence from Dublin in support of 'Dr. Campbell's observation that insanitary surroundings have probably much less direct influence upon puerperal mortality than is generally supposed ... unless infection is introduced from without'. It agreed that 'the problem with which the country is faced is rather one of organisation and education than of principles directly concerned with current obstetric practice'.

The Lancet also agreed on the importance of antenatal care. Identifying problems early was clearly preferable to dealing with complications during a home birth, but this would be effective only if midwives and general practitioners were properly trained. *The Lancet* was 'in absolute agreement with Dr. Campbell in aiming at the total abolition of the so-called handy woman, and with the suggestion that there should be much closer cooperation between the doctor and the trained midwife'.

Dame Janet reported that only 50–60% of births were conducted by midwives and that these had a lower mortality rate than when a doctor was involved. Often a doctor was 'summoned merely to apply forceps with the sole object of expediting the labour', and this was when the problems began. The doctor's antiseptic precautions were usually inadequate and her report gave detailed advice on this. A major reason for the high intervention rate was pain. A doctor could give chloroform but a midwife was not allowed to administer any kind of pain-relieving drug.

Specialist opinion

Specialist obstetricians agreed with Dr Campbell but their perspective was narrower than hers. In 1919 Victor Bonney, a pioneer of gynaecological surgery, wrote that the delivery room in the woman's home should be converted into an operating theatre, with meticulous asepsis, a dedicated anaesthetist and a nurse to assist the obstetrician. This was hopelessly impractical but his description of the perfunctory antiseptic technique of the single-handed obstetrician/anaesthetist rang true.

Specialists also criticised excessive intervention by general practitioners (GPs) and the disorganised state of antenatal care – and the inadequacy of their own midwifery fees, which made them focus on gynaecology rather than obstetrics. Even so, very few women could afford them. At a meeting of the

Medical Women's Federation in 1925 one member spoke of 'the gap between conditions in the practice of specialists and those which obtained in, for example, the East-End of London'. For the vast majority of women, if medical help was needed it came from a GP relying on his undergraduate training which, all agreed, was pitifully inadequate.

Questions in Parliament

Dame Janet's report recommended 'investigation by the medical officer of health of all maternal deaths due to childbirth, and of all cases of puerperal infection, whether fatal or not'. This could be organised by the Ministry of Health. However, the report also observed that 'the establishment of a comprehensive and efficient maternity service is largely a matter of administration and finance'. That would need government support.

The report was echoed by more calls for action. In 1925 the Midwives' Institute passed a resolution asking the Ministry to ensure that every maternal death was followed by an autopsy and a full investigation, and that notification of birth should include the name of the person who actually delivered the baby. The Institute wanted the annual reports of the medical officers of health to distinguish between cases involving a midwife and those involving a doctor. Clearly relations between the professions were still problematic.

Dr Ethel Cassie, Chief Medical Officer for Child Welfare in Birmingham, noted the high mortality from puerperal sepsis and the 'considerable disagreement as to its nature, its evidence, and as to the methods of prevention'. She urged the development of a national maternity service with approved midwives and 'a panel of obstetric surgeons with special training and experience'. She also pointed out the needs for better nursing care in the puerperium and better antenatal care.

In 1925 a question about deaths in childbirth was raised in Parliament. Minister of Health Neville Chamberlain replied that a circular had already been issued in 1924 urging local authorities to provide more maternity beds and to respond to the reports of their medical officers. He 'saw no need for special investigation on this point'. More pressure was needed but one-third of women in the UK still did not have the vote and the Equal Franchise Act of 1928 was still three years away. As in 1907, the pressure would come from extra-parliamentary action. This time it would involve the highest women in the land.

Lucy Baldwin and the National Birthday Trust Fund

One of those women was Lucy Baldwin, the wife of Prime Minister Stanley Baldwin. She became the vice chair of the National Birthday Trust Fund, established in 1928 to provide pain relief for women during labour. She also established 'Mrs Stanley Baldwin's Anaesthetics Appeal Fund' in 1929, with the aim of developing affordable forms of pain relief to be administered by midwives in the mother's home. The ban on midwives giving analgesia, which had led to so much unnecessary intervention, did not end until the Midwives Act of 1936.

Born in Bayswater in 1869 and raised in Sussex, Lucy Baldwin played cricket in her youth for 'The White Heather Club', one of the first women's teams. In 1892 she married Stanley Baldwin. She was 'the more ambitious of the two'. They had seven children, the first of whom was stillborn, and all Lucy's labours were long and painful. Maternity care was her main focus. Her work contributed to The Midwives' Act and inspired the funding of The Lucy Baldwin Maternity Hospital in Stourport-on-Severn, which opened in 1929 and closed in 2006. The National Birthday Trust Fund continued as a leading charity and made important contributions to perinatal research before joining with Birthright in 1993.

A message from the Queen

The year 1928 was a landmark year in the campaign for safer childbirth. On 28 February Westminster Central Hall (by then the biggest meeting hall in London) was the scene of what the BMJ called 'a very largely attended meeting to discuss maternal mortality'. One difference from the 1907 meeting in Caxton Hall was that almost all the attendees were women. Another was that the social spectrum was broader. A message was read from the Queen.

> Her Majesty views with grave concern the continued high rate of maternal mortality, and feels that a very real endeavour should be made to remove this reproach from the national life ... The Queen trusts this may be achieved through the education of mothers themselves in the need for ante-natal care, through inquiry into the immediate causes of mortality in childbirth, and through a wider provision of first-rate medical and midwifery services.

The message was a succinct summary of Dame Janet Campbell's recommendations. How the Queen came to know about them is unclear.

Queen Mary had an austere image but she was a mother (see Figure 2.3). She had had six babies and her youngest son, born after a difficult labour, had died at the age of 13. It is unclear who organised the 1928 meeting and invited her to contribute, but Dame Janet was one of the speakers and the chair was Dame Edith Lyttleton, one of the first people honoured when King

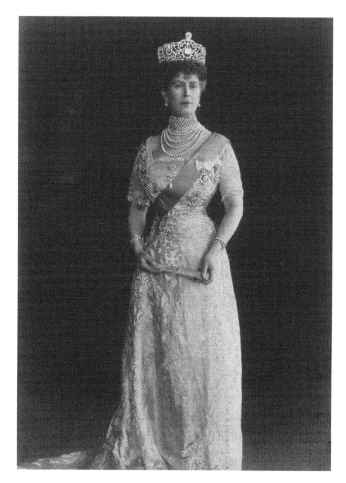

Figure 2.3 Mary of Teck (1867–1953), Queen Consort 1910–36

George V founded the Order of the British Empire in 1917. Dame Edith had been appointed Dame Commander of the Order for her work among refugees.

Her Majesty's intervention had a powerful effect. The meeting unanimously carried a comprehensive resolution which was conveyed to the Ministry of Health. On 15 May 1928 Neville Chamberlain announced a 'scheme by which local medical officers of health will inquire into the circumstances of every death during childbirth and practitioners will be asked to supply information to the Ministry'. This was the forerunner of the Confidential Enquiry into Maternal Deaths (CEMD).

Chamberlain also announced two new Ministry of Health committees. One would consider the training and working conditions of midwives. The other, chaired by Sir George Newman, would 'advise upon the application ... of the medical and surgical knowledge at present available, and inquire into the needs and direction of further research work'. Dame Janet Campbell would be a member of both.

The Maternal Mortality Committee

In the same year two veteran activists, May Tennant and Gertrude Tuckwell, formed the unofficial Maternal Mortality Committee. It represented a wide range of voluntary groups, including the National Birthday Trust Fund and the Women's Cooperative Guild. It held its own conference in Westminster Central Hall on 30 October 1928, attended by Sir George Newman and 'many hundreds of women, representing societies and municipal organizations concerned with work amongst mothers and infants'. Its stated aim was to check on progress since the previous conference in February.

Neville Chamberlain addressed the meeting and 'exhorted the gathering to "patience and courage" – a phrase which', said The Lancet, 'evoked some sharp comments from his feminine critics afterwards'. Delegates criticised his inadequate spending on milk for infant welfare clinics. He replied that this was 'due to the prolonged industrial disturbance of 1926 [i.e. the General Strike] which seriously reduced the national revenue'.

Dr Marion Philips reported that she had investigated how well local authorities were following the Ministry's recommendations. Out of 127 county and borough councils, 116 had replied, of which 61 were 'putting into force half or more of the provisions for which a grant in aid could be obtained'. She added that 'it was not the richest areas which were, in general, doing most'. Dr Philips was a Doctor of Science from the London School of Economics and the Chief Woman Officer of the Labour Party. In 1929 she was elected as an MP for Sunderland and became Britain's first Jewish woman MP.

Another radical who addressed the meeting was Dora Russell, named in The Lancet as Mrs Bertrand Russell. She said that in Germany, where miscarriages were notifiable, 40–50% of all pregnancies had ended in miscarriage in 1926. The economy had collapsed from war debts and women were resorting to abortion. 'No enquiry into maternal mortality', she said, 'could be blind to the alternatives either of legalizing abortion or of providing proper contraceptive measures at clinics'. The Lancet reported that this statement 'was received with loud applause from a section of the conference and no audible dissent'.

The meeting passed a resolution welcoming the new departmental committees and the voluntary committee kept a watchful eye on them until it disbanded in 1935. The legalisation of abortion in Britain is discussed in Chapter 8.

Scotland's first Report

Scotland had the same high rate of maternal mortality as England but the country had its own department of health. Since 1885 it had been governed by the Scottish Office, and in 1919, when the Ministry was established in England, the Scottish Board of Health was set up.

In 1917 Britain's first enquiry into individual maternal deaths was begun in Aberdeen by Matthew Hay, the medical officer of health. He asked local registrars to notify him of deaths of women during pregnancy or within four weeks after childbirth. Further details were obtained from the midwife or health visitor working in the district. In 1923 a preliminary report on these enquiries was sent to the Scottish Departmental Committee on Puerperal Mortality and Morbidity, which reported in 1924 that 'puerperal mortality is but a section of a much wider group of causes of puerperal morbidity'. It concluded that the solution lay in the improvement and extension of maternity services and paying particular attention to puerperal sepsis.

An analysis of 252 maternal deaths in Aberdeen in 1918–27 was published in 1928. It included a special census of births in the city in 1924, allowing rates to be calculated by the woman's age, parity and social circumstances. This method was then applied to the whole of Scotland, where the 2,527 maternal deaths between 1927 and 1932 were compared with data collected about all 39,205 births occurring in the country in one 6-month period. This use of control groups remains unique and never became part of subsequent maternal mortality enquiries in either Scotland or England.

The Departmental Committee

In England, a major step forward came in June 1928 when the Departmental Committee on Maternal Mortality and Morbidity was established, chaired by Sir George Newman. It included Dame Janet Campbell, Dr Ethel Cassie and Sir Walter Fletcher FRS, the secretary of the Medical Research Council (MRC). It also had professors of obstetrics and gynaecology from London, Manchester, Sheffield and Newcastle; medical officers of health from Newcastle and Wiltshire; a doctor from the East End Maternity Hospital and two pathologists, one of them Leonard Colebrook, the MRC bacteriologist who features in Chapter 5. The status and expertise of its membership, drawn from across the country, demonstrate the priority now being given to maternal mortality. The British Medical Association (BMA) was not officially represented but had agreed to co-operate.

A National Enquiry

The Departmental Committee set out to enquire into individual maternal deaths across England and Wales. A form was designed, with the agreement of the BMA, and issued to local authorities. When a maternal death occurred, the local medical officer of health had to fill in all the available information and send the form in confidence directly to the Ministry. The reports were then scrutinised and classified by two relatively junior obstetricians, G. F. Gibberd, then a registrar at Guy's Hospital, and Arnold Walker (later Sir Arnold), an assistant obstetric surgeon at the City of London Maternity Hospital.

These two scrutinisers were asked to divide the deaths into those directly due to childbearing (more than a third of which were due to puerperal sepsis) and those not primarily due to pregnancy. Importantly, they were to look for 'the primary avoidable factor'. This system set the pattern for the Confidential Enquiries for the rest of the century and beyond.

The Interim Report

By 30 April 1930 a total of 3,079 reports had been received – about two-thirds of all the maternal deaths in England and Wales. The Departmental Committee decided they were representative and issued an interim report in 1930 based on the first 2,000 cases. Of these, 1,596 were directly due to pregnancy and 404 were due to a disease which may or may not have been made worse by pregnancy – mainly diseases of the heart and lungs.

Of the pregnancy-related deaths, 38.6% were due to sepsis. The report devoted 16 pages to this condition, with detailed advice about its prevention. Interestingly, however, as shown in Figure 2.4, the chapter on sepsis was preceded by one on abortion, which caused 10.5% of the deaths. The Committee did not comment on 'the sociological effects of abortion or birth control', but found no evidence for current public alarm that the incidence of abortion was increasing. Other chapters discussed antenatal care, the use of anaesthetics and analgesics and medical education.

Chapter 8 discussed 'a national maternity service'. The Committee did not 'consider it within their province to express an opinion on the best method of financing it', but they said it should 'make provision for all persons not in a position to procure for themselves similar benefits by private arrangement'. They set out plans in some detail. They said 'the provision of facilities for specialist help and advice in difficult cases is one of the great needs of an improved service' and suggested that 'the services of consultants might be

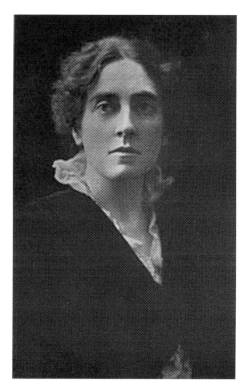

Figure 2.4 May Tennant (1869–1946)

made available by special local arrangements for all small Maternity Homes and Hospitals'.

In short, this remarkable report represented a unique combination of carefully compiled facts and imaginative recommendations – what we would today call 'blue sky thinking'. Many of its ideas would eventually become reality in the form of the NHS. It took evidence from a wide range of witnesses and organisations, including the Midwives' Institute and the newly established British College of Obstetricians and Gynaecologists, founded in 1929.

One of its 11 appendices included a note from Sir George Newman emphasising that 'all information given on the Inquiry Form will be treated as *strictly confidential*'. Most members of the Departmental Committee were doctors, and confidentiality had always been at the heart of medical practice. Facts could therefore be revealed to them without fear of reprisal and no names or places would be identified when the reports were published. This would remain a permanent feature of the Confidential Enquiries and was the basis for their accuracy and effectiveness.

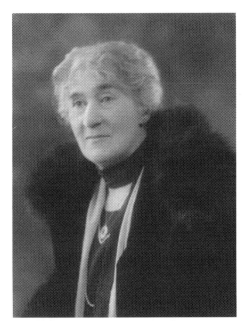

Figure 2.5   Gertrude Tuckwell (1861–1951)

The Final Report

The final report, published in 1932, covered 5,805 deaths and developed the recommendations further. It included descriptions of the maternity services of the Netherlands, Denmark and Sweden, and a review of research, particularly work on the streptococcus by Leonard Colebrook. Other chapters focussed on maternal morbidity and on areas of England with high maternal mortality, investigated in a separate report by Janet Campbell, Isabella Cameron and Dilys Jones.

The Departmental Committee recommended that enquiries should continue on a routine basis. The Ministry of Health asked medical officers of health to continue sending reports on a revised and shortened form. G. F. Gibberd and Arnold Walker continued their work of assessing the reports, and summary statements were included in the *Chief Medical Officer's Annual Report* from 1932 to 1953. Similar systems continued in Wales, Scotland and Northern Ireland.

The 'Rochdale Experiment'

Meanwhile, at least one local medical officer of health was taking action without waiting for national guidelines. Maternal mortality was highest in

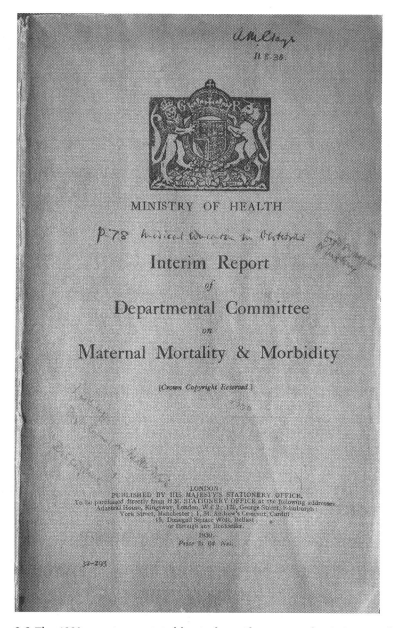

Figure 2.6 The 1930 report, annotated by Andrew Claye soon after being appointed a part-time professor of obstetrics at Leeds University. He became the president of the Royal College of Obstetricians and Gynaecologists in 1957 and was knighted in 1960.

DEPARTMENTAL COMMITTEE ON MATERNAL
MORTALITY AND MORBIDITY

INTERIM REPORT

TABLE OF CONTENTS

CHAPTER I – INTRODUCTION

CHAPTER II – REPORT OF MATERNAL DEATH
INVESTIGATION

CHAPTER III – ABORTION IN RELATION TO MATERNAL MORTALITY

CHAPTER IV – PUERPERAL SEPSIS

CHAPTER V – ANTENATAL CARE

CHAPTER VI – THE USE OF ANAESTHETICS AND ANALGESICS
IN OBSTETRIC PRACTICE

CHAPTER VII – MEDICAL EDUCATION IN OBSTETRICS

CHAPTER VIII – REPORT ON A NATIONAL MATERNITY SERVICE

CHAPTER IX – CONCLUSIONS AND RECOMMENDATIONS

Figure 2.7 The contents page of the 1930 interim report

the industrial areas of the north of England, and the Lancashire town of Rochdale, as mentioned earlier in this chapter, had the unenviable distinction of having the highest maternal mortality rate in the country. When Dr Andrew Topping arrived there in 1930 as a medical officer of health he was shocked by this statistic. Aged 40, he, after serving in the First World War, had studied public health in his home city of Aberdeen, which had recently published its own census of maternal deaths.

As the medical officer of health in Rochdale, he was in charge of the town's antenatal clinics but – as he later admitted – he knew next to nothing about pregnancy care. He soon realised that he was not alone. His ignorance was shared by his fellow doctors and by the women of Rochdale, who 'were intensely keen to be told the truth about conception, pregnancy and confinement in simple, straightforward language'. He noted that the local doctors had various theories about the reasons for the high maternal mortality but 'careful examination of the individual case reports showed that none of these suggestions could hold water'. The real reasons were lack of antenatal care and excessive intervention in labour.

Topping's approach was to tell the truth to the doctors and the women, frankly and without any recrimination. Twice-weekly meetings were held by organisations, including the churches and the cooperative society, to explain the purpose of antenatal care and the benefits of letting nature take its course rather than imploring a doctor to hurry the birth along. The local newspaper, *The Rochdale Observer*, gave the fullest help 'without any scare headlines or alarmist paragraphs'. The leaders of the BMA division, the Midwives Association and the health committee gave 'very cordial help' but the key step was informing the women. 'They knew what a proper ante-natal examination connoted and any doctor or midwife who scamped it was very soon talked about, greatly to his or her prejudice.'

Within two years the maternal mortality rate in Rochdale was halved, and when Dr Topping moved on, the improvement was maintained by his successor, Dr Innes. In 1935 a team of obstetricians reported this success in the BMJ. They commented on the mutual cooperation among everyone involved and the provision of information to the public, adding, 'It is important to observe that the results were obtained by a change of spirit and method and without any alteration in the personnel or any substantial increase in public expenditure.'

Dr Topping was a remarkable man. He became the director of the London Ambulance Service during World War II and worked for the United Nations, afterwards becoming the first professor of social and preventive medicine at the University of Manchester and the president of the Society of Medical Officers of Health. His landmark achievement, however, was the 'Rochdale Experiment', which needed the skills of diplomacy and leadership as well as breadth of vision, and had far-reaching effects across the country. As Sir George Godber commented many years later:

> *All this procedure had been intended to do was to secure improvements by the local review of cases, but it was soon apparent that avoidable factors were too often present in antenatal and intranatal care for the opportunity for central remediable action to be ignored. This led to the decision to undertake a national confidential enquiry.*

Problems continue

In other places, however, change was slow. In 1934 the Ministry of Health sent officials to areas with high mortality and a sample of areas with low mortality in order to review maternity services and socio-economic conditions.

Individual deaths were studied in detail. The reports also studied abortion, a major cause of maternal death which was widely discussed at the time, including in a report published in 1939 by the Interdepartmental Committee on Abortion (see Chapter 8).

The General Register Office, using data from death registration, provided much more detail about maternal mortality than was normal in its other publications. This revealed a surprising and disturbing pattern, tucked away in a report with an unremarkable title. The *Registrar General's Supplement on Occupational Mortality* showed a reverse social class gradient in maternal mortality, suggesting that the medical care of pregnant middle-class women at this period was more dangerous than that available to working-class women, who were looked after mainly by midwives.

Change at last

The maternal mortality rate started to decrease in Scotland in the early 1930s and elsewhere in the United Kingdom in the mid-1930s. The change is usually attributed to dramatic improvements in therapy – the introduction of sulphonamides to treat sepsis and blood transfusion to treat haemorrhage (see Chapters 5 and 6). However, the fall in mortality in both England and Scotland began just before these major breakthroughs, and it seems likely that better organisation of maternity care and changes in practice were already starting to make a difference. The effect of the new antibiotics in particular was dazzling, but it should not blind us to the major contribution made by the painstaking work described in this chapter. Those reports were just as revolutionary in their own way and had a lasting effect in improving maternity services and transforming the safety of childbirth.

3 HOW THE CONFIDENTIAL ENQUIRIES EVOLVED

In July 1949 the twelfth British Congress of Obstetrics and Gynaecology was held in the Friends Meeting House in Euston Road, London. Ten years had passed since the eleventh Congress and much had happened in that time. War had come and gone, the National Health Service (NHS) had been founded, and obstetrics and gynaecology had become an established specialty. The 1949 Congress was opened by Minister of Health Aneurin Bevan and chaired by Sir Eardley Holland, the immediate past president of the Royal College of Obstetricians and Gynaecologists (RCOG).

The final session on the Friday afternoon was a discussion on maternal mortality. It was led by the RCOG president, Sir William Gilliatt, who was nearing the end of his term of office. In a few months' time Hilda Lloyd (later Dame Hilda) of Birmingham would become the RCOG's first female president. Gilliatt, a Lincolnshire farmer's son, was a consultant at King's College Hospital London and in 1952 he would be appointed the surgeon-gynaecologist to the Queen.

The mood of the discussion could well have been one of self-satisfaction. Britain's maternal mortality rate had fallen by 75% – from 4.4 per 1,000 births in 1928 to around 1 per 1,000 in 1948 – and antibiotics had all but abolished the historic scourge of puerperal fever. But instead the Congress focussed on what still needed to be done. Medical officers of health across England were sending the Ministry of Health (MoH) confidential reports on individual maternal deaths and a 'primary avoidable factor' was being identified in almost 50% of cases.

A new system

At that time the *Journal of Obstetrics and Gynaecology of the British Empire* (later the *BJOG*) devoted at least 50 pages of each issue to a 'Review of the Current Literature' – papers mainly from Europe with a translated summary, and some from the USA. Among the American papers were reports of maternal death investigations by local committees of experts who decided to publish their findings. This approach was discussed at the twelfth British Congress, as described later in the first Confidential Enquiry into Maternal Death (CEMD) Report:

> *Sir Eardley Holland suggested to the Minister of Health the possibility of adopting a similar method of investigation in this country. Consultations followed with the Royal College of Obstetricians and Gynaecologists and with the Society of Medical Officers of Health, resulting in the adoption of a new system of enquiry designed to bring in all who might contribute information – family doctor, medical officer of health, midwife and, in all cases, consultant obstetrician. The arrangements came into operation at the beginning of 1952.*

The RCOG already had a good relationship with the MoH. Aneurin Bevan is often perceived as establishing the NHS against medical opposition, but he had the support of the RCOG. Eardley Holland, the son of a Surrey rector, had worked with the pioneering epidemiologist Dr Janet Lane-Claypon in the 1920s on her study of perinatal deaths. During the war he organised the evacuation of pregnant women from London and then worked with the MoH on the planning of maternity services for the new NHS. This was some years before they became part of Bevan's portfolio.

Sir George Godber

With Bevan at the MoH was another country lad who rose to the top in medicine and indeed became one of the most influential British doctors of the twentieth century. George Godber, the son of a Bedfordshire market gardener, won scholarships to Oxford and the London Hospital Medical School. When he graduated in 1933 he was determined not to practise in any system where patients had to pay – a view reinforced by working as a general practitioner (GP) in the East End of London. He did that while studying for qualifications before joining the MoH in 1939. He too helped to organise maternity services for evacuees and worked on plans for the new NHS.

He supported the Confidential Enquiries throughout his long career at the MoH. He became Chief Medical Officer (CMO) in 1960, was knighted in 1962 and retired in 1973 as the century's longest-serving CMO – and, many believe, the best. Despite opposition he campaigned against smoking and made the contraceptive pill free on prescription. In 1950 he suggested that midwives should be an official part of the Confidential Enquiries, but this idea was ahead of its time. It was eventually implemented in 1990. Godber lived to be 100, so he was able to send the director of the Enquiries a handwritten letter of congratulation.

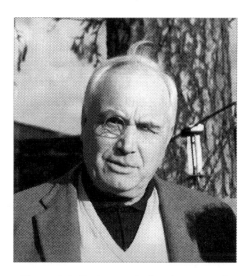

Figure 3.1 Sir George Godber (1908–2009)

How the system worked

Before 1950 maternal deaths were investigated by local medical officers of health, who gathered information and sent it direct to the MoH. They were advised to 'seek the assistance of a consultant or specially qualified practitioner in cases of unusual difficulty' but rarely did so. Under the post-1950 system of Confidential Enquiries, when a maternal death occurred they would inform a local consultant obstetrician and give him what information they had. The consultant would then 'obtain full clinical information about the case – as far as possible by personal enquiry from those who have been in attendance on the woman, whether hospital staff or family doctor'.

Another innovation was the appointment of regional assessors, 'a senior obstetrician of high standing in the area of each Regional Hospital Board', who would receive the obstetrician's report and the medical officer's comments and could ask for further details. He (initially all were men) would then add his views about the cause of death and any avoidable factor, either clinical or administrative, and send the report to the CMO. The regional assessors met once a year for a confidential discussion of the material they received.

Although midwives were not formally involved, they were consulted, as was the Royal College of Midwives. Arrangements were also discussed with the RCOG and the BMA, but, as Sir George Godber wrote later, 'always in an informal way. It was probably that informality that made the scheme work with minimal objection.'

Arnold and Joe

The MoH's two consultant advisers on obstetrics made the final assessment and classification – a job they had already been doing for many years. One of them was Arnold Walker, who had been one of the young medical examiners for the departmental report of 1932. By 1952 he was a consultant at the City of London Maternity Hospital and the chairman of the Central Midwives Board. A Yorkshireman from a long line of family doctors, he helped to advance the position of midwives and was much loved for his common sense, as noted in his obituary by Sir George Godber in the *British Medical Journal* (BMJ) of 28 September 1968, which included his photograph. He became Sir Arnold in 1966.

The other was Arthur Joseph 'Joe' Wrigley, born in Lancashire and another down-to-earth northerner. He studied medicine at St Thomas's Hospital, London, became head of its Department of Obstetrics and was awarded the CBE in 1965. His name is well known to obstetricians because he designed forceps small enough to be used safely by non-experts. When he died in 1983

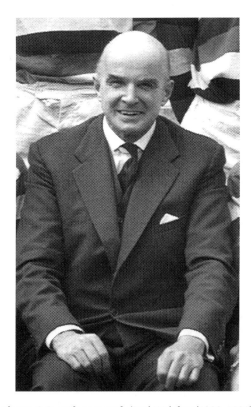

Figure 3.2 Arthur Joseph 'Joe' Wrigley (1902–1983)

Godber wrote in the BMJ about his 'sound sense, humanity, and utter lack of pretension' and gave an insight into how the Enquiries began.

He and the late Arnold Walker were the real founders of the Confidential Enquiry into Maternal Deaths . . . It was largely due to trust in Arnold and Joe that the inquiry was accepted in 1952 almost universally in the specialty and indeed the medical and midwifery professions. The form of the inquiry was worked out in long discussions with the two consultant advisers. With Katherine Hirst they drafted the chapters of the report and then discussed it at meetings with the regional assessors and with Dr Martin, the statistician. We all had considerable anxiety about publication of the first report with its acknowledgment of inadequacies in the services, but public acceptance of the honesty and value of the profession's intentions soon allayed that.

Today it is hard to imagine such a warm relationship between the public, the MoH and the profession, but it was crucial to the early success of the Enquiries. Another surprising feature of the first Report is its small team of authors. There were only five, two being Drs Walker and Wrigley. Dr Katherine Hirst was a senior medical officer at the MoH (appointed OBE in 1958), and Dr W. J. Martin was the statistician. The fifth author was Dr Archibald Marston, consultant anaesthetist at Guy's Hospital, London, and foundation dean of the Faculty of Anaesthetists. He had helped to drive the development of anaesthesia as a specialty, but he too was known for his 'loyalty, honesty and modesty'.

The authors' reputation for integrity inspired trust from doctors around the country. The first Report commented that 'in the majority of cases frank and detailed reports are received and frequently it is clear that only an investigator who is an expert in the field will be aware of all the points on which enquiry is needed'. The Enquiry also benefitted from Regional Assessors' wide experience and local knowledge, but the Report emphasised that anonymity was essential: 'Names of attendants are not required and it is the pooled information obtained over a period of years that provides the basis of the present report.'

The Enquiry, the first-ever nationwide professional self-audit, remains a shining example which has been hard to replicate (see Chapter 16). Its benefits were being felt even before its findings were published. The 1952–4 Report commented that everyone involved, 'however experienced he or she may be . . . benefited from their educative effect'.

Avoidable factors

Prior to the Enquiry 'avoidable factors' had been identified by the medical officer of health, but under the new system the local consultants and the regional assessors were asked to give their views. Not surprisingly, their standards varied. They had differing opinions about the treatment of specific conditions and the criteria for choosing home or hospital delivery. It was up to the consultant advisers to achieve a balance reflecting 'the most generally accepted standards of good antenatal and obstetric care . . . which might be expected from any doctor with a continuing interest in midwifery or from any well-trained midwife'.

Practice guidelines were still many years in the future, but some official advice on standards had been published, including a memorandum on antenatal care from a Standing Maternity and Midwifery Advisory Committee – which happened to be chaired by Arnold Walker. As consultant adviser he took account of this, but nonetheless 'practical and generally accepted standards, attainable under average practice conditions, have been applied rather than ideal'. Women were expected to take some responsibility, but 'in no case has a patient's refusal to accept termination of pregnancy or to practise contraception been regarded as an avoidable factor'. The Report also emphasised that an avoidable factor did not mean that death could certainly have been prevented. It was 'an indication that the risk of death could have been, at least, materially lessened'.

The first Report

The first CEMD Report, covering the years 1952–4, was published in 1957. Sir George Godber commented: 'If the delay seems long, it was partly due to the time lag in collecting all the reports and partly to trepidation about outside reaction to the confidentiality enforced. In the event, there was no public criticism on either of these grounds.'

The Report itself was a slim volume of 60 pages, published by Her Majesty's Stationery Office at three shillings and sixpence (18p). It had 10 chapters and a detailed appendix. The first chapter gave the background, methods and overall figures. There had been 1,094 deaths due directly to pregnancy or birth, and 316 deaths from associated causes. Of the direct deaths, more than half were due to three conditions – toxaemia of pregnancy, haemorrhage and pulmonary embolism – each of which had its own chapter.

Surprisingly perhaps, sepsis did not. Puerperal sepsis, the leading cause of maternal death until the 1930s, caused only 42 deaths in 1952–4, though infection was still a problem. It accounted for 91 deaths associated with abortion, which did have its own chapter. Counting the sepsis deaths in that chapter was a bold decision which had far-reaching consequences (see Chapter 8) because it confirmed that abortion, with a total of 153 deaths, was one of the leading causes of maternal mortality.

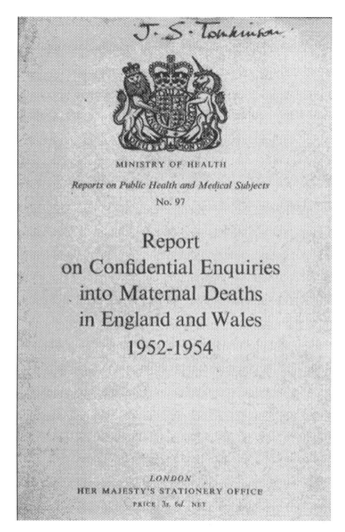

Figure 3.3 The first CEMD Report, property of J. S.Tomkinson FRCOG, Consultant at Guy's Hospital, London, and Secretary General of the International Federation of Gynaecology and Obstetrics

Cardiac disease caused 121 deaths, which were classified as 'associated with pregnancy' (see Chapter 10). The overwhelming majority were due to the after-effects of rheumatic fever, a common streptococcal throat disease in the early twentieth century which could damage the heart valves. This chapter warned that the damage is progressive, so a successful birth early in life is no guarantee of safety in a later pregnancy.

There was a chapter on caesarean section, which was associated with 183 deaths, many of them due to the condition that had led to the operation. At that time only 3% of births in England were by caesarean section but, then as now, the rate was hotly debated. According to a separate chapter anaesthesia accounted for the deaths of 49 women, only 13 of whom had had a caesarean section. Twenty-five of the women who died after general anaesthesia had had a forceps delivery, and the commonest cause of death was inhalation of stomach contents. The frequent use of general anaesthesia for vaginal birth was why the Report's panel of authors included a specialist anaesthetist from the start (see Chapter 11).

Avoidable factors were identified in 406 deaths and discussed in chapter 9. In 120 cases the responsibility was judged to lie wholly with the GP, in 101 with the hospital medical staff, in 96 with 'the patient' and in 14 with the midwife. Often, however, it was shared. No names or places were identified either publicly or privately and the original reports were destroyed after the Report was written. The final chapter summarised the recommendations for improving care but it also acknowledged that in the current state of medical knowledge some deaths were unavoidable.

The reaction

Official reports often gather dust, but the first CEMD Report attracted immediate attention. In August 1957 a *Lancet* editorial began by pointing out how often an avoidable factor had been identified and then homed in on the Report's main finding – that 'the greatest source of error was inefficient or insufficient antenatal supervision ... many doctors and midwives do not yet appreciate when a materially increased risk to the mother is present'. *The Lancet* concluded that deaths could be prevented by:

(1) *better antenatal care, especially in the early detection and early treatment of toxaemia;*
(2) *prompter and more efficient treatment of haemorrhage, especially through the use of flying squads for emergency and domiciliary midwifery; and*
(3) *better selection of cases for specialist care in hospital, especially women in the older age-groups and higher parities.*

Having its messages disseminated in this way by medical journals was exactly what the CEMD needed, and it set the pattern for the future. From 1957 onwards Reports were published at intervals of three years, which gave enough time for changing patterns to be recognised. The 'triennium' remained

THE LANCET

LONDON: SATURDAY, AUGUST 24, 1957

Prevention of Maternal Deaths

THAT childbirth is far safer now than it was twenty years ago is well known. The extent of the improvement is evident from the maternal mortality : whereas in 1934 there were 2880 maternal deaths in England and Wales, in 1954 there were only 480. Almost as remarkable as the reduction in numbers has been the alteration in the causes of death. In the

Figure 3.4 Leading article in *The Lancet*

the basis for CEMD Reports until 2008. If the Reports had been annual they would have had repetitive recommendations. The three-year interval gave them more impact.

Even so, when the Report for 1955–7 appeared in 1960 the overall messages were largely unchanged, though the number of deaths, particularly from haemorrhage, had fallen. Once again a *Lancet* editorial conveyed a sense of urgency about the need to pay attention to avoidable factors, but it would take years to change practice across the country.

The Cranbrook Report

Meanwhile there were other official reports on the maternity services. In 1953, after the Conservatives returned to power, the government invited an economist, C. W. Guillebaud (great-uncle of the contraception expert John Guillebaud), to chair a committee of enquiry into the NHS. Some feared that this might lead to its being completely dismantled, but the committee recommended little change apart from increased spending on hospitals. It noted, however, that division of the service between the three separate parts of the NHS – hospitals, general practice and local health authorities – was preventing effective cooperation between midwives, GPs and obstetricians, and it asked for something to be done about that.

Another committee was set up, chaired by Lord Cranbrook, which made wide-ranging recommendations. It wanted GPs to take charge of the antenatal clinics run by local authorities. It suggested that only GPs who had done appropriate training should be on the 'obstetric list' (which paid extra fees) and that hospital beds for confinement 'should, where possible, be GP beds'. Today, however, the Cranbrook Report of 1959 is remembered only by advocates of home birth because it recommended that there should be enough hospital beds for 70% of all confinements.

The Peel Report

Similarly, the Peel Report of 1970 is still blamed for sounding the death knell of home births in Britain. In reality, the trend was well under way in 1967 when the Department of Health set up a committee to consider the future of domiciliary midwifery. Its members, who included the president of the Royal College of Midwives, elected Sir John Peel as their chairman. Peel, a Yorkshireman, was surgeon-gynaecologist to the Queen and, as president of the RCOG, had persuaded it to support the 1967 Abortion Act (see Chapter 8).

The committee took evidence from many organisations and its report was 135 pages long. Paragraph 277 read: 'We consider that the resources of modern medicine should be available to all mothers and babies and we think that sufficient facilities should be provided to allow for 100% hospital delivery. The greater safety of hospital confinement for mother and child justifies this objective.'

That last sentence has since generated much debate, but it reflected the mood of the times. In 1970 *The Lancet* commented: 'The goal of 100% deliveries

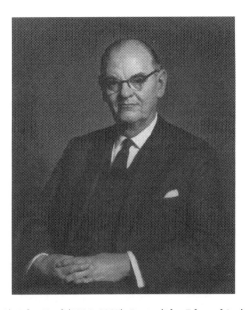

Figure 3.5 Sir John Peel (1904–2005). Portrait by Edward Irvine Halliday

in hospital will appeal to most doctors because of its promise of increased safety, and to the public because socially the trend is overwhelmingly towards regarding hospital as the right place for delivery.'

The first 30 years

Against this changing background, the CEMD continued through the 1960s and 1970s with its 16 regional assessors (all of them leading obstetricians with national reputations) and its small team of central assessors. Arnold Walker and Joe Wrigley retired from that role in 1964 to be replaced by senior figures who in turn gave way to others of similar professional stature. The anaesthetic assessor from 1955 to 1972 was Geoffrey Organe, who became Sir Geoffrey in 1968. His successor, Gordon Robson, was knighted in 1982. From 1976 onwards the team included a pathologist, the first being Professor Ian Dawson from the new medical school at Nottingham.

The format of the Reports changed little over those years. Initially a chapter was devoted to each of the four main causes of maternal death (see Chapters 6–9), with the others being grouped together. In 1961–3 new chapters were introduced, including one on amniotic fluid embolism, a recently recognised condition in which the lungs are damaged by fluid from the uterus escaping into the bloodstream. The 1964–6 Report introduced a chapter on sepsis, which, despite the optimism of the 1950s, would continue to be a problem from then on (see Chapter 5).

The proportion of deaths with avoidable factors did not fall. Indeed, by 1976–8 it had increased to 58%. This did not mean that maternity care had worsened, however. As standards of care rise, more and more avoidable factors are identified. In 1979–81 the term was changed to 'substandard care', which could include administrative factors and resources as well as clinical factors.

The 1982–4 Report was the last for England and Wales. It included a retrospective review by Sir Alexander Turnbull, a professor at Oxford who was the lead obstetric assessor at that time. He noted that the maternal mortality rate (MMR) had halved every 10 years since the Enquiries started and commented that 'the marked reduction in deaths from hypertensive disease and haemorrhage might have occurred simply because it was easy to improve on poor previous standards of care'.

He also pointed out that the introduction of contraception, sterilisation and safe abortion in the 1960s had reduced the birth rate, particularly at the extremes of reproductive life when the mortality rate is at its highest, and he ended by looking forward to a continuing halving of the MMR in future decades – a prediction which was to prove over-optimistic.

The Enquiry expands

From 1985 onwards the CEMD covered the whole of the United Kingdom. Scotland had been publishing its own reports at varying intervals between 1965 and 1985, the last covering both maternal and perinatal deaths. Northern Ireland had produced reports at 4-year intervals from 1956 to 1967, but the falling numbers of deaths made anonymity hard to maintain and the interval increased to 10 years. The same problem applied in Scotland, where there were only 14 maternal deaths in 1971. A UK-wide Enquiry allowed all four countries to participate in the CEMD process while preserving anonymity. (Similar logic led to the Republic of Ireland joining the Enquiries in 2009.)

The team expanded considerably. Each of the four nations contributed its own Department of Health representative, statistician and assessors in obstetrics, anaesthetics and pathology, and each of the 14 English regions had its assessors in obstetrics, anaesthetics and pathology, as did Scotland. Even without the presence of midwives, the 1985–7 UK Report had an editorial board with 24 members and observers, and acknowledged the contribution of no fewer than 64 regional and Scottish assessors. The Editorial Board was chaired officially by a Deputy Chief Medical Officer but in practice by the chair of the Clinical Sub-Group, Professor Vic Tindall of Manchester for 1985–7 and Professor Bryan Hibbard of Cardiff for 1988–93.

Radical change would come in 1994, but the first three UK-wide Reports followed the pattern of the previous reports for England and Wales. One innovation was a new chapter on 'early pregnancy deaths', which replaced the chapters on ectopic pregnancy and abortion. There had been no deaths from illegal abortion since 1982. The UK Reports still had a chapter on 'late' deaths (more than 42 days after delivery), but it was small because the English assessors had decided in 1984 to stop investigating these deaths. It soon became apparent that this was a mistake – for example, suicides from postpartum depression were being missed (see Chapter 12) – and it was decided in future to investigate deaths up to six months after birth, or later at the discretion of the assessor.

Times change

The Report for 1991–3 came at a time of profound change in the patterns of disease, in medical treatment and in the politics of maternity care. The number of indirect deaths (due to medical conditions worsened by pregnancy) was rising and would soon exceed the number of direct deaths (see Chapter 10). The Enquiries appointed a medical assessor, Dr Michael de Swiet, author of *Medical Disorders in Pregnancy*, which was (and still is) the standard textbook on this subject. He continued as medical assessor for 17 years, coping with a steadily increasing workload singlehandedly until 1999, when he was joined by Dr Catherine Nelson-Piercy.

Intensive care was also becoming more important. In the 1991–3 Report, 104 of the 228 women who died had been admitted to an intensive care unit. A new chapter on this emerging specialty was written by Dr Sheila Willatts. She was the anaesthesia assessor for England, and, as well as being a consultant anaesthetist in Bristol, she was a pioneer of critical care and a past president of the Intensive Care Society, which she and others had founded in 1970.

The most radical change came in 1989, when the science of maternity care was revolutionised by a new book, *Effective Care in Pregnancy and Childbirth*. The editors were Iain (later Sir Iain) Chalmers, Murray Enkin and Marc Kierse. Chalmers, the son of an obstetrician, was the director of the National Perinatal Epidemiology Unit in Oxford and the founder of the Cochrane Collaboration. He and his colleagues brought maternity care into the era of evidence-based medicine, which challenged its reliance on traditional teaching. Practice in future would be based wherever possible on statistically sound clinical trials.

Traditional maternity care was also challenged in 1993 by the report of the Expert Maternity Group chaired by Baroness Julia Cumberlege, Parliamentary Under-Secretary of State at the Department of Health. Entitled *Changing Childbirth*, it aimed to give women more choice in maternity care and to place more responsibility on midwives. The RCOG was excluded from the Group's deliberations and the tone of the Group's report was seen as confrontational by many obstetricians, who feared it would recreate the old division between obstetricians and midwives.

The CEMD Report for 1991–3, published in 1996, commented in its preface: 'Given the greater emphasis on team working, and following the implementation of *Changing Childbirth*, we are pleased that for the next Report we will have the benefit of Regional and Central assessors in midwifery.' The first midwifery assessors were Mrs N. R. Shaw and Mrs Kathryn Sallah.

Emerging issues

As well as responding to change, the Enquiries were themselves leading the way. The 1991–3 Report included a new section on postnatal depression, suicide, substance abuse and domestic abuse written by Dr (later Professor) Gwyneth Lewis, a Principal Medical Officer at the Department of Health. She joined the Enquiries in 1992 and she appointed the first psychiatric assessor, Dr Channi Kumar, who drove the expansion of the Enquiry into mental illness until his untimely death in 2000. He was replaced by Dr Margaret Oates

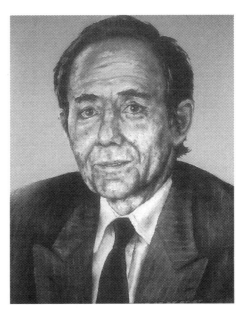

Figure 3.6 Prof. Channi Kumar (1938–2000). Portrait by Patrick Weiss. By permission of the Institute of Psychiatry

(see Chapter 12). Between them they were responsible for the growth of the sub-specialty of perinatal psychiatry, which many believe arose from the early work of this Report.

Dr Lewis, a consultant public health physician with a special interest in women's health, went on to become the director of the Enquiries and led them through a major period of change recorded in the Reports from 1994–6 to 2006–8. She developed a parallel focus on the medical, social and other factors which lay behind the vast inequalities identified in these Reports, with poorer health outcomes for mothers from ethnic minority groups and those who lived in poorer social circumstances – factors which often occurred together.

She also improved the presentation of the Reports with an A4 format, a picture on the cover and a new title, 'Why Mothers Die', designed to attract attention. The name succeeded in doing so and was continued for the next two Reports. In 2003 Dr Lewis changed it to 'Saving Mothers' Lives' to reflect the real purpose of the Enquiries – not just to record cases, but also to learn lessons, make recommendations and have them implemented, so that the subsequent outcomes for women would be entirely different.

Persuading the doubters

In the early 1990s there was a prevailing view among some administrative and medical personnel at the Department of Health that the Enquiries had served their purpose, now that the numbers of maternal deaths in the UK had fallen to a low level. Dr Lewis defended them and saved the day. The Enquiries' findings, particularly in relation to totally unacceptable inequalities, remained alarming, and the Reports came more and more to the notice of the media, parliamentarians and the professions. Every three years the Report's publication day was covered in the national news and statements in Parliament. The need to continue was explained in the 1994–6 Report, published in 1998:

> *The task now is to improve results that are already very good . . . We have to make these improvements while continuing to ensure that for the majority of women pregnancy and childbirth remain as natural and enjoyable as possible. Maximum safety does not mean unnecessary medicalisation. The increasing role of evidence-based practice should help to ensure that only effective interventions are used but when it comes to rare catastrophes, scientific data may be lacking. This Report therefore represents a blend of clinical experience and evidence-based recommendations.*

The doubters were also persuaded by the wider public health focus Dr Lewis brought to the Enquiries. The 1997–9 Report revealed a shocking 20-fold difference in the risk of death between the least and most disadvantaged groups in British society. The 2000–2 Report highlighted the facts that one third of the women who died were clinically obese, that the MMR was three times higher in women from ethnic groups other than white, and that mortality rates are particularly high among refugees and asylum seekers (see Chapter 13). These issues continued to cause public concern for the next 20 years, and they are still far from resolved.

The role of the Director

The 1994–6 Report continued the panels of central and local assessors but introduced a new nomenclature. Dr Lewis was the director, and an obstetrician, Professor James Drife of Leeds, was the clinical director. Although obstetric analysis was still at the heart of the Enquiries, the public health aspects had greatly increased, making the director's role more important and more challenging. Gwyneth Lewis became the 'tsar' of maternity services in the Department of Health and, while continuing to be actively involved in the CEMD, she was responsible, among many other things, for policies to improve the quality of maternity services in England. *Maternity Matters* and *National Service Framework for Maternity Services* were just two of the resulting publications, which were quickly followed by the other home nations.

Being at the centre of the data and evidence, Professor Lewis was able to use the latest CEMD findings to defend, input or develop national policies or guidelines with the sole aim of improving maternal and newborn care. As director, she was allowed complete independence to express her views, and those of the CEMD authors, freely and without fear of government censure of any kind. This is quite different from similar enquiries elsewhere, especially in South Africa, as recounted by its former director, Professor Bob Pattinson (see Chapter 15). Such freedoms are essential but sadly are no longer the case in the UK now that the Enquiries have been moved to agencies at arm's length.

Reorganisation and the future

Until 1998 all government reports were published by Her Majesty's Stationery Office, which became The Stationery Office after privatisation in 1996. The Report for 1997–9, however, was published by RCOG Press on behalf of the National Institute of Clinical Excellence (NICE), which was formed in 1999 as part of the Department of Health and Social Care. Further changes followed. NICE created a new organisation, the Confidential Enquiry into Maternal and Child Health (CEMACH), which was the publisher of the next two Reports; CEMACH then became the Centre for Maternal and Child Enquiries (CEMACE), which published the Report for 2006–8.

Remarkably, Dr Lewis kept her team of assessors together through these high-level reorganisations, each of which brought the Enquiry under renewed scrutiny. One aspect that came under threat was the use of anonymised case histories, or 'vignettes', in the Reports. Clinicians have always learned from individual cases and these vignettes drove home the messages in a memorable way. The directors vigorously defended them and they survived, though much reduced in number. Their anonymisation required considerable editorial skill and no case was ever correctly identified from the published reports.

The Reports retained their basic structure with chapters devoted to specific conditions, but the 2000–2 Report introduced a chapter on 'Issues for Midwives' and the 2003–5 Report added one on 'Issues for General Practitioners', as well as an introductory chapter on 'Top Ten Key Recommendations'. This included an urgent call for national guidelines on the obese pregnant woman, sepsis, and pain and bleeding in early pregnancy.

The arrival of the Internet in the late 1990s changed the way professionals and the public find information. *Why Mothers Die 2000–02* and *Saving Mothers' Lives* (the 2003–5 Report) are easily found online and are freely accessible. The 2006–8 Report was published as a supplement to the *British Journal of Obstetrics and Gynaecology* (BJOG 2011;18:Suppl 1) and quickly became a basic reference in the global scientific literature. The effect of the communication revolution has been dramatic, and 10 years on the Report for 2006–8 is still cited in research papers on an almost daily basis.

The CEMD is now established in its new home, the National Perinatal Epidemiology Unit in Oxford, where it is part of MBRRACE-UK, as described by Professor Marian Knight in Chapter 14. Its reports are published annually in hard copy and free online.

The first 60 years

How did the CEMD survive six decades of profound change in public attitudes and government policy with its basic principle, confidentiality, intact? It was because only the investigations were confidential. The facts were published for all to see. Far from being a 'cover-up', the CEMD involved public exposure of shortcomings at all levels, with constructive advice on how to put things right. Only the names were missing and no lawyers were ever involved. The public as well as the professionals understood that, if confidentiality were breached, this altruistic process would have to end. The radical idea proposed 'with trepidation' in the early 1950s seemed to strike a chord with everyone and continues to save lives in the twenty-first century.

4 THE MISSING CHAPTER? PROLONGED LABOUR AND OBSTETRIC TRAUMA

Across the globe the 'big five' causes of maternal death are haemorrhage, toxaemia, abortion, sepsis and obstructed labour. The Confidential Enquiry into Maternal Deaths (CEMD) Reports of the 1950s had chapters on the first three of these. Sepsis did not have its own chapter because at that time people thought infection had been vanquished by antibiotics. But the shadow of the streptococcus still lingered in the long-term effects of rheumatic fever (which attacks the heart valves), and the Report for 1952–4 had a chapter on cardiac disease – as did all subsequent Reports.

That first Report had 10 chapters, including one on pulmonary embolism, one of the leading causes of maternal death in England and Wales. Of the remaining five, one explained the method of the CEMD, another summarised all the avoidable factors and the final chapter discussed the Report's overall conclusions. The other two chapters covered caesarean section and anaesthesia. Caesarean section was associated with 183 deaths, many of them due to the underlying complications that had led to the operation. Another 49 deaths were attributed to anaesthesia, which was often used in those days for forceps delivery.

Unsurprisingly then, the early Reports focussed on the major concerns of the time. From today's perspective it is surprising that these did not include the complications of vaginal birth. We know that difficulties in labour and birth are a major problem in developing countries. In the 1950s they were still common in England and Wales.

Complications of childbirth

They were listed in the early Reports as an appendix which gave all causes of maternal death using terminology specified by the Registrar General (RG). Six of those causes related to prolonged labour or obstetric trauma, as shown in Table 4.1.

Apart from 'rupture of the uterus' (included as a separate chapter from 1955 onwards), none of these terms has a precise definition. 'Other trauma' and 'other complications' are uninformative, and 'disproportion' is notoriously

Table 4.1 Complications of childbirth: 1952–1975

Delivery complicated by …	1952–1954	1955–1957	1958–1960	1961–1963	1964–1966	1967–1969	1970–1972	1973–1975
Abnormality of the bony pelvis	5	3	1	1	-	-	-	1
Disproportion or fetal malposition	22	30	30	29	34	5	10	14
Prolonged labour of other origin	42	16	18	6	15	4	10	14
Other trauma	55	40	46	43	29	-	2	1
Other complications of childbirth	66	42	44	54	42	21	7	5
Rupture of the uterus	-	33	-	38	30	18	12	11
TOTAL	**190**	**164**	**139**	**171**	**150**	**48**	**41**	**36**

difficult to define. All we really know is that all these deaths were associated with vaginal birth, and that, when added together, they outnumbered the deaths associated with caesarean section.

Deciding the Cause of Death

The terminology came from the International Classification of Disease (ICD), which dates from the nineteenth century. In 1893 an international congress in the USA adopted a nomenclature proposed by a French physician, Jacques Bertillon. The terms changed as medical knowledge advanced, and from 1900 onwards the ICD was revised at approximately 10-year intervals. The sixth revision (ICD6) was published in 1949 by the recently formed World Health Organization. The ICD is used mainly by public health doctors and epidemiologists, and the extent of obstetric input into ICD6 is unclear.

By using this terminology in its appendix the CEMD could compare its figures with those of the RG, whose data came from death certificates. Certification had existed in the UK since 1837, and it was up to the doctor who signed the form to decide what to write under 'cause of death'. As the *British Medical Journal* (BMJ) noted in 1952: 'The introduction of the international form of death certificate has caused little change in existing practice in England and Wales, where an almost identical certificate had already been in use since 1927.'

By contrast, the CEMD's data came from the forms sent to the Enquiry. The RG and CEMD figures were listed side by side in the appendix, and the numbers often differed. The CEMD had better information, but the RG had more cases in the early years, when not all deaths were reported to the Enquiry. The figures in Table 4.1 are from the CEMD.

Unsatisfactory as the ICD6 terminology was, it gives us a picture of the stage that obstetric practice had reached in the 1950s and is worth looking at in more detail.

'Abnormality of the Bony Pelvis'

This term dates from the nineteenth century, when rickets was common in British cities and severe distortion of the pelvis was a major obstetric problem. In 1884 a survey in Clydeside found signs of rickets in every child examined. In London's Great Ormond Street Hospital one in three children showed some features of the disease. Severe rickets causes the growing pelvis to collapse, leading to dwarfism. The baby's growth is unaffected, making normal birth impossible. The first-ever caesarean section in Glasgow Maternity Hospital was performed on Catherine Colquhoun in 1888, and soon afterwards two similarly afflicted women underwent this new procedure (Figure 4.1). Without it their babies would have certainly have died and they would probably have died too.

Contracted pelvis

After lack of sunlight was identified as the cause of rickets in the 1920s the incidence fell. Children got opportunities to experience sunshine and were given cod liver oil and other vitamin D supplements. By the 1950s rickets had almost disappeared and major pelvic abnormality was rare in women, but obstetricians remained concerned about minor pelvic abnormality. What that actually meant, however, was unclear. A national meeting held in London to discuss 'minor degrees of contracted pelvis' failed to agree on a definition.

In 1954 a leading obstetrician, Sir Hector MacLennan of Glasgow, spoke to the BMA's annual meeting about 'contracted pelvis'. It had accounted for 27% of admissions to Glasgow Maternity Hospital in 1903 and 4% in 1954. The degree of contraction had also become much less severe and Sir Hector

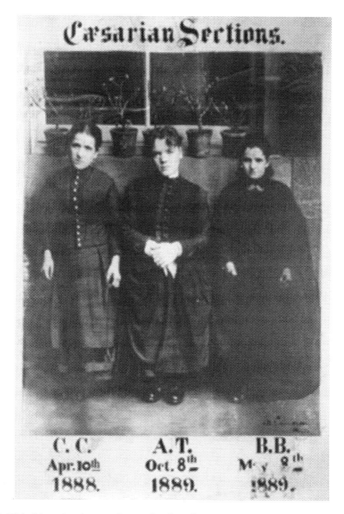

Figure 4.1 This historic picture shows the first three women ever to undergo caesarean section in Glasgow Maternity Hospital, and the dates of their operations. Catherine Colquhoun is on the left. The window sill behind them is about one metre high.

advocated 'trial induction' of labour before term, with recourse to caesarean section only if necessary.

'Trials of labour' often ended in forceps delivery. Sir Hector reported that, when it was carried out for contracted pelvis, the fetal loss rate was 11.4%. That figure, unconscionable today, was a considerable advance on the early twentieth century, when craniotomy had often been necessary to achieve delivery. ('Craniotomy' means using a destructive instrument to crush the baby's head.) In Glasgow craniotomies outnumbered caesarean sections until 1908.

In 1954 Glasgow Maternity Hospital's caesarean section rate for contracted pelvis was under 2%. This was in line with figures elsewhere. Figures from Aberdeen show that in 1952 the overall caesarean section rate was 2.2% in the city and under 1% in the rest of the region.

Sir Hector acknowledged that by 1954 caesarean section had become safer than in the past but nonetheless he concluded: 'Let us prevent this operation from falling into disrepute and becoming the first resort of the lazy obstetrician, the escape of the timid obstetrician, and the cloak of the incompetent.'

Similar but less grandiloquent warnings about caesarean section were being made elsewhere, including Edinburgh, where contracted pelvis had caused four maternal deaths every year in the city's main maternity hospital during the 1920s but none after 1945. By then the incidence of contracted pelvis was under 3% and vaginal birth was achieved in more than 50% of cases. Even so, two craniotomies were carried out in Edinburgh after 1950.

'Disproportion'

In the 1950s the term 'contracted pelvis' was being replaced by 'cephalopelvic disproportion' (CPD). The idea that the baby's head is too big to pass through the mother's pelvis is easy to understand, but the reality is difficult to predict. In 1953 G. F. Gibberd (one of the young scrutineers in the 1928 Enquiry and later a leading London obstetrician) wrote about disproportion in an American journal. He concluded that it is easy to tell when CPD is *not* present, but a prediction of CPD was likely to be right 'about 50% of the time' and 'the cost of a mistake is generally an unnecessary caesarean section'.

In 1949 Professor Chassar Moir of Oxford wrote in the BMJ about pelvimetry and cephalometry – measurement of the pelvis and the baby's head during pregnancy. At the end of the nineteenth century clinical pelvimetry had been 'an essential part of every obstetrical examination'. This required internal examination via the vagina but in the 1930s the obstetricians' fingers were being replaced by radiography. In some hospitals X-ray pelvimetry became a routine part of antenatal care in a first pregnancy, and Professor Moir believed the trend would continue into labour itself. In the 1950s, however, X-rays in pregnancy were linked to childhood leukaemia, and by the 1960s it was clear that radiology was of little practical help in cases of suspected minor disproportion.

'Fetal Malposition'

Malposition refers to the position of the baby's head during labour. At the end of pregnancy the head only just fits into the maternal pelvis and during labour the baby has to manoeuvre its way through. At first it looks to one side. When it reaches the mid-pelvis, which is circular in cross-section, the head can begin to turn. At the end of labour the baby is facing backwards, towards the mother's sacrum. It then lifts its head while passing under her pubic arch. Usually the shape of the pelvis makes these positional changes happen naturally, but sometimes the baby's head faces the wrong way or turns in the wrong direction.

Sometimes malposition can be corrected by the fingers of the obstetrician or midwife, but more often a special instrument is needed. Normal forceps are dangerous in such cases. They are curved to fit the shape of the pelvis and should only be used when the baby's head is facing the sacrum. Trying to use them to rotate the baby's head can damage the vagina and cause catastrophic bleeding. Straight forceps for rotation were introduced in 1916 by Christian Kjelland, a Norwegian obstetrician, but it takes time to learn how to use them safely. A vacuum extractor developed in the 1950s by Tage Malstrom, a Swedish obstetrician, can correct some types of malposition but did not become popular in the UK until the 1990s.

Standard forceps can also cause severe haemorrhage if a doctor tries to apply them before the cervix is fully open – an error with potentially disastrous consequences. A tear in the cervix can easily extend upwards and involve the uterus. Checking for full dilatation may be difficult and requires experience. In the 1950s more than 50% of all births took place outside hospital, but it was hard for general practitioners to gain this experience. Even in hospital, junior doctors were sometimes left to cope without adequate supervision.

'Prolonged Labour'

The phrase 'prolonged labour' first appeared in a medical journal in 1948 in a report of a labour lasting six days. In 1949 H. L. Sheehan, originally from Glasgow but by then a professor of pathology in Liverpool, reported 147 autopsies of women in Glasgow who had died from 'obstetric shock' after labours lasting more than 48 hours. Obstetric shock resembles the shock that results from severe haemorrhage, but it can occur after a long labour without bleeding. Prolonged labour is often due to disproportion and all the babies in Sheehan's report had weighed more than 9 pounds (4.1 kg).

In 1952–4 prolonged labour caused the deaths of 42 women in England and Wales. Today it seems unthinkable that this could happen in a developed country, and even then it was hard to believe. In 1961 Professor Norman Jeffcoate of Liverpool wrote in *The Lancet*: 'Many of us are old enough to remember the time when a serious disturbance of uterine activity in the first stage of labour nearly always resulted in the death of the baby, and sometimes of the mother as well.' He implied that this was a distant memory, but this was less than a decade after the 1952–4 CEMD Report.

In the 1960s labour was defined as prolonged if it lasted for more than 24 hours. Causes of slow labour were said to be 'inco-ordinate uterine action', 'hypotonic inertia', 'hypertonic inertia', 'uterine exhaustion' or minor degrees of pelvic contraction. Doctors adopted a hands-off approach, fearing that amniotomy (rupture of the membranes) might introduce infection and that powerful uterine stimulants might make matters worse. Pain relief in a first labour took the form of heavy sedation with morphine or heroin.

Preventing prolonged labour

In 1969 this cautious approach was challenged by a groundbreaking report in the BMJ entitled 'Prevention of prolonged labour'. In Dublin the National Maternity Hospital had introduced a policy of active management of labour. This involved amniotomy and oxytocin infusion (an intravenous 'drip'), but only after vaginal examination had confirmed that labour had started, and only in women having their first baby.

Professor Kieran O'Driscoll and his colleagues reported the success of this policy in 1,000 consecutive labours and drove a coach and horses through current obstetric thinking. They attacked as fallacies the idea that there were

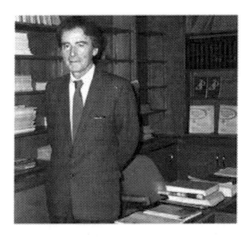

Figure 4.2 Kieran O'Driscoll (1920–2007). This photograph was taken by Professor Tom Baskett in Halifax, Nova Scotia, and appears in his book *Eponyms and Names in Obstetrics and Gynaecology*, along with a fuller description of how Professor O'Driscoll changed women's experience of labour.

different types of uterine malfunction and that a prolonged first labour was often due to disproportion. Slow labour was actually due to inadequate production of oxytocin by the woman's pituitary gland and could be restored to normal by giving an identical hormone through a drip.

For some obstetricians this paper was a revelation. Others saw the policy as dangerously interventionist. Advocates of natural childbirth objected to the whole idea of labour being 'managed' by obstetricians. Interestingly though, the paper began with the woman's point of view:

> *Prolonged labour presents a picture of mental anguish and physical morbidity which often leads to surgical intervention and may produce a permanent revulsion to childbirth, expressed by the mother as voluntary infertility … The harrowing experience is shared by relatives, and by doctors and nurses to the extent that few complications so tarnish the image of obstetrics.*

Contraception was illegal in Ireland at that time, adding poignancy to the words 'voluntary infertility', but women in many countries would surely have empathised with these words.

The policy led to less intervention at the end of labour – in the National Maternity Hospital the caesarean section rate was 4% and Kjelland's forceps were famously banned from the building. Obstetricians from the UK were slow to appreciate these benefits, but a watered-down version of the policy eventually changed obstetric practice in Britain and the USA. Nevertheless, times change. In 2017 the caesarean section rate for first-time mothers in Dublin's National Maternity Hospital was 29% – similar to the current rates in other hospitals in the British Isles and elsewhere.

'Rupture of the Uterus'

Rupture of the uterus was not part of ICD6, but it was a chapter in the CEMD Reports in 1955–7 and from 1961–3 to 1982–4. Over that time the picture changed considerably. In 1955–7, 8 of the 33 deaths were due to spontaneous rupture after repeated labours over many years in older women. Two of the women were having their eleventh baby and one each their tenth, ninth, eighth, sixth, fifth and fourth. Other deaths were due to obstructed labour or medical intervention, sometimes in a home birth or in a small maternity home.

Because older women with many children were particularly at risk, the 1961–3 Report strongly recommended that age and parity should be taken into account when deciding the place of birth. It also noted that some deaths from uterine rupture 'were associated with the administration of oxytocic drugs'. Oxytocin is safe when given intravenously in a first pregnancy but dangerous in a highly parous woman, and, when given by mouth in the form of 'buccal pitocin', its effects are unpredictable.

Again in the 1964–6 Report some of the women who died had received oxytocic drugs, either in hospital or in a general practitioner (GP) unit. Attempts at forceps or assisted delivery caused 12 deaths, 8 of them in hospital. In the next Report, however, deaths from traumatic rupture fell sharply and the total fell to 19. Oxytocic drugs were involved in 6 cases.

Deaths from trauma almost disappeared in the 1970s and the total number of deaths from rupture of the uterus continued to fall steadily, with most cases still involving oxytocin. In 1982–4 three deaths were reported, and thereafter the chapter was replaced by one on genital tract trauma, in which the total remained in single figures.

'Other Trauma' and 'Other Complications of Childbirth'

Until 1966 at least 50% of the deaths in Table 4.1 were under the unhelpful headings 'Other trauma' or 'Other complications'. This was frustrating for the CEMD assessors, who introduced a chapter on 'Sudden death in labour' in 1955–7. In it they complained that post-mortem examination had often amounted to 'an almost perfunctory search for the cause of death'. They wrote that after a sudden death the coroner may order an autopsy by a forensic pathologist who is not experienced in obstetric work and 'the results are often less helpful and sometimes quite useless for the purposes of this enquiry'.

Of the 44 sudden deaths in the new 'Sudden death' chapter, 17 were due to obstetric shock, 11 to amniotic fluid embolus and 9 to air embolus. Obstetric shock occurred after prolonged labours at home, in small maternity homes and in hospital. Amniotic fluid embolus is an unpredictable condition even today. Air embolus was a complication of criminal abortion. The chapter also included deaths after forceps delivery and in the 1958–60 Report it was replaced by a chapter on 'Obstructed and assisted labour'.

That chapter noted that assisted delivery had been involved in 115 deaths but it focussed on the 43 deaths from definite obstruction, all but 10 of which had occurred in a homebirth or a GP maternity home. The detailed descriptions of obstetric manoeuvres by inexperienced doctors made harrowing reading. The chapter concluded that 'by far the most important avoidable factor was the making of an unwise arrangement for a confinement to take place in the patient's own home or in a Maternity Home'.

'Arrangements for Confinement'

In the 1958–60 Report another new chapter appeared, headed 'Arrangements for confinement'. It began by acknowledging that comments in earlier Reports about 'unwise arrangements' had been too vague to be helpful. 'If insufficient emphasis on the importance of sensible arrangements for the confinement has been made in the past, an attempt will now be made to correct this omission.' It then gave detailed examples of 10 cases in which death could have been avoided by hospital booking, and a list of five criteria for booking a birth at home or in a GP maternity home.

In the next Report the chapter analysed deaths according to the planned place of birth. The total number of deaths in 1961–3 was 936. Of these, 194 women had been booked for home birth and 96 for a GP unit. No booking arrangements had been made for 218 women. In the home birth group the leading cause of death was pulmonary embolism and in 29 of the 37 cases pre-existing venous thrombosis had been noted. Those women had therefore been at high risk. Other causes of death included toxaemia and heart disease, for which home birth was clearly inappropriate.

The chapter continued through the 1960s and 1970s. By 1967–9 home births accounted for less than 10% of the total number of deaths. The 1970–2 Report, however, painted a worrying picture. Across England and Wales 10.4% of births had taken place at home, but 18% of the maternal deaths were of women booked for birth at home or in a GP unit, and in half of those cases avoidable factors had been present.

In 1973–5 things changed dramatically. The total number of deaths fell by almost a third to 390, among which only 10 women had been booked for home birth and 38 for a GP unit. Many of them had correctly been transferred to hospital booking. The numbers were similar in 1976–8. By then 98% of births in England and Wales were in hospital and the chapter on booking arrangements was discontinued.

The change in the 1960s

A striking feature of Table 4.1 is the step change between 1964–6 and 1967–9. After remaining static for years, deaths from complications of childbirth suddenly fell by two-thirds, from 150 to 48. This was not due to a dramatic increase in the national caesarean section rate, which was 3.4% in 1964 and 4.4% in 1969, or in the hospital caesarean section rates, which rose from 4.4% in 1964 to 5.9% in 1969.

There must be other reasons for this dramatic reduction in deaths. The most obvious is that general practitioner obstetrics was at last being taken seriously.

Some credit for this must go to the CEMD for highlighting the death rate in home births and GP units in the 1950s, and giving clear booking criteria in the 1958–60 Report.

That CEMD Report, published in 1963, was followed in 1964 by a series of articles in the BMJ headed 'Obstetrics in General Practice'. Between March and July the journal published a weekly series of 21 articles by the leading obstetricians of the day, writing in collaboration with general practitioners. They covered every aspect of obstetrics from antenatal care and education to toxaemia, normal labour and neonatal care. The final articles were entitled 'Home or hospital?' and 'Equipment for domiciliary obstetrics'.

'Home or hospital?' was written by Professor (later Sir) John Stallworthy of Oxford (father of the poet Jon Stallworthy). In 1937 he had been tasked by his predecessor, Professor Chassar Moir, with setting up the Oxford obstetric flying squad. In 1939 he was invited by the Regius Professor of Medicine, the marvellously named Sir Farquhar Buzzard, to take charge of a new 'area department' bringing GP obstetricians into a closer relationship with the hospital.

Stallworthy's article, and all the others in the BMJ series, showed a sympathetic understanding of the problems GP obstetricians faced. There was no undercurrent of competition or blame. Stallworthy looked forward to the day when the choice of place of birth would not be restricted by lack of hospital maternity beds, which he described as a 'crisis'. The choice, he said, lay with the woman, helped by advice from her GP. What was essential, he added, was a good relationship between the midwife, the GP and the consultant.

So, was there a 'missing chapter'?

Looking carefully at the complications in childbirth in the 1950s makes it easier to understand why they were not lumped together in a single chapter in the CEMD Reports. From a twenty-first-century perspective almost all of those deaths could have been prevented by timely caesarean section but, in the 1950s, a national caesarean section rate of 25% (as it is now in the UK) would have seemed ridiculous. The Reports took a down-to-earth approach to 'avoidable factors' and made sure their recommendations were practical and realistic. The chapters on 'Obstructed labour' in the 1950s and 'Booking arrangements' in the 1960s came at the right time, achieved their purpose and then quietly disappeared as new concerns emerged.

5 HOW THE CHANGE BEGAN: THE STORY OF SEPSIS

Infection of the uterus is rare in the non-pregnant state and during pregnancy because the cervix is closed and a plug of mucus keeps vaginal bacteria out. For a few days after birth, however, the cervix remains open and the raw area where the placenta was attached inside the womb is vulnerable to germs. But even then, infection occurs only if new bacteria from outside the body are introduced by poor hygiene or a failure of aseptic practice.

Childbed fever, or puerperal sepsis, was the most feared complication of pregnancy during the nineteenth and early twentieth centuries, when it accounted for almost half of all maternal deaths. After antibiotics were developed the incidence fell dramatically, so much so that in early Confidential Enquiry into Maternal Deaths (CEMD) Reports sepsis did not merit its own chapter. Infection had not gone away, however. A chapter first appeared in the 1964–6 Report and has featured in all the Reports since.

In 2006–8 sepsis was again the leading cause of direct maternal death, though the numbers were an order of magnitude smaller than in the 1930s. In the 2020s the COVID pandemic has been another reminder that infection will always be with us. Our recent experience shows parallels with the first recorded account of epidemic puerperal sepsis, published by Alexander Gordon in 1795.

Alexander Gordon of Aberdeen

Gordon, a graduate of Aberdeen University and the medical schools of Edinburgh and Leiden, spent five years as a naval surgeon before studying midwifery in London. He returned to Aberdeen in 1785. Four years later the city was struck by an epidemic of childbed fever and another followed in 1792. Gordon closely observed them both and wrote a treatise which he dedicated to Thomas Denman, who was his teacher in London and had been a pupil of William Smellie (see Chapter 1).

Gordon's conclusions were far ahead of their time. During the eighteenth century it was believed that infection was caused by miasma – 'something in the air' – but Gordon wrote:

The cause was not owing to a noxious constitution of the atmosphere, for if it had been it would have seized women in a more promiscuous and indiscriminate manner. But this disease seized such women only as were visited, or delivered by, a practitioner or a nurse who had previously attended patients affected with the disease.

This was the first description of the infectious nature of childbed fever. Gordon went further and gave the first advice on how to prevent the infection spreading: 'The patient's apparel and bed clothes ought to be burnt or thoroughly purified; the nurses and physicians who have attended patients affected with puerperal fever ought carefully to wash themselves and get their apparel properly fumigated before it be put on again.' And, he admitted, 'It is a disagreeable declaration for me to mention, that I myself was the means of carrying the infection to a great number of women.'

He advertised his treatise for sale in the local paper, but it did not bring him the gratitude he expected. This is hardly surprising because he included the names of the practitioners and nurses who had carried the disease. His new ideas did not go down well with his colleagues or the general public and he had to leave the city. He returned to the navy, contracted tuberculosis and died at his brother's farm near Aberdeen in 1799.

The death of Mary Wollstonecraft

Two years after Gordon published his treatise, Mary Wollstonecraft died of puerperal sepsis in London. Her tragic case history, summarised in what follows, is all the more shocking because she was a healthy and fiercely independent woman. One of Britain's leading literati, she had written an eyewitness account of the French Revolution. She published *A Vindication of the Rights of Woman* in 1792 and is now regarded as the founder of modern feminism (Figure 5.1).

In 1797 she had had one normal pregnancy and was looking forward to having her second baby at home. She had no intention of 'lying in' after the birth, but she did book a midwife, Mrs Blenkensop. Labour started on 30 August and the baby, a girl, was born at 11.20 p.m. The first sign of trouble was that the placenta did not follow. After three or four hours Mrs Blenkensop called Dr Poignard, a physician-accoucheur at Westminster Lying-in Hospital. It took him several hours to remove the placenta and there was severe blood loss.

The next day Mary was 'remarkably well', but on 3 September she started to have shivering fits followed by high fever. This continued for three days, when she became 'surprisingly better' only to deteriorate shortly afterwards. Usually

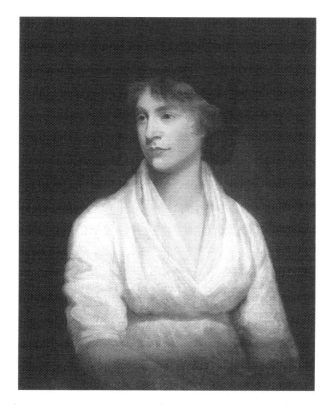

Figure 5.1 Mary Wollstonecraft (1759–97). Portrait by John Opie

death follows rapidly, but she resisted for another three days before succumbing on 10 September.

The baby, also named Mary, grew up to be equally talented. During her childhood she visited her mother's grave regularly and at the age of 16 she eloped with the poet Percy Shelley. At 19 she wrote the classic novel *Frankenstein*. It involves a scientist bringing a dead creature to life and was partly inspired by her early bereavement.

Lying-in hospitals

Mary Wollstonecraft's death was presumably caused by Dr Poignard's attempts to remove an abnormally adherent placenta – a rare condition that is very difficult to treat even now. It may or may not be relevant that both he and Mrs Blenkensop came from a hospital. Lying-in hospitals had been introduced in the middle of the century, first in Dublin with the foundation of the Rotunda in 1745, and shortly afterwards in London, where the Westminster

Lying-In Hospital was founded in 1752. Living conditions in the slums of both cities were appalling and such charitable institutions offered women somewhere clean to give birth.

It soon became evident that, despite their best intentions, lying-in hospitals were susceptible to outbreaks of puerperal fever. In London the overall maternal mortality rate in the eighteenth century was around 1.5%. In the lying-in hospitals it could suddenly rise to 4% or more and remain at that level for weeks or months before falling again just as suddenly. There is no evidence of an outbreak at Westminster Lying-in Hospital in 1797, but sporadic cases occurred and aseptic practice was still far off in the future.

Erysipelas in Abingdon

The earliest report of an epidemic of puerperal fever in England was in Abingdon, Berkshire. It was linked to erysipelas, a cellulitis of the superficial layers of the skin caused by the streptococcus – the same organism that causes puerperal fever. There is a fiery red rash and infection can spread to deeper layers, causing a rapidly progressive fasciitis which can be fatal. In 1813 cases of erysipelas were reported in villages near Abingdon. They included a 12-year-old boy who had to have both legs amputated to save his life, and there were two deaths and two cases of puerperal fever. In Abingdon itself 20 cases of puerperal fever were reported, almost all fatal, and many nurses developed erysipelas of the arms. The epidemic ceased in September 1814 and was reported in one of the emerging journals of the time.

Controversy in the United States

In America isolated epidemics of erysipelas were reported in small towns in the 1840s and 1850s and were often associated with fatal puerperal fever. The disease was recognised as contagious. In 1844 a report in the *American Journal of Medical Science* stated that it was 'unquestionably communicated by individuals, whether physician or nurse, who have been much with the disease, to women at or immediately after childbirth'.

In Philadelphia in 1840 it had a disastrous effect on one of the city's respected general practitioners, Dr Rutter. Seventy of his patients developed puerperal fever and two died. Other doctors had no cases or very few. Dr Rutter quarantined himself, washed thoroughly, shaved his face and head, and changed all his clothes and equipment, even his pencil. He resumed work after several weeks, but puerperal fever still followed him everywhere and he was forced to leave the city.

In Boston in 1843 an up-and-coming physician, Oliver Wendell Holmes Sr, published a paper on 'The Contagiousness of Puerperal Fever'. He later became famous as a poet and writer. In fact, it was he who coined the word 'anaesthesia', in a letter to William Morton, the American dentist who first gave ether to a patient in 1846. Because of his fame Holmes has been widely credited as the first to recognise that puerperal fever is contagious, but, in his report, he himself gave credit to Alexander Gordon.

Holmes was only 34 when he published his paper. It was bitterly attacked by a senior academic, Professor Charles Meigs of Philadelphia, for daring to suggest that a medical man could do harm to his patients. Holmes responded calmly when challenged but, nonetheless, when writing about puerperal fever, he did not mince his words: 'The existence of a private pestilence in the sphere of a single physician should be looked on not as a misfortune but a crime.' He meant that a doctor who recognised that he was a carrier should stop practising obstetrics.

Outbreaks in Ireland

Morton's report of ether anaesthesia in 1846 was followed a year later by the discovery of chloroform anaesthesia in Edinburgh. It made James Young Simpson a national hero. He too recognised that puerperal fever was contagious. In 1850 he wrote: 'I believe that patients during labour may be locally inoculated with a *materies morbi* capable of exciting puerperal fever [and] that this is liable to be inoculated by the fingers of the attendant.'

The cause remained a mystery, however, and outbreaks within lying-in hospitals continued. When registration of deaths was introduced in England and Wales in 1837 the hospital records could be compared with national data. In England the overall maternal mortality rate was 4 per 1,000 births. In the Rotunda Hospital Dublin, which had kept meticulous records since its foundation, outbreaks had occurred about every 10 years, pushing the rate up to 40 deaths per 1,000 births or even higher.

Semmelweis in Vienna

In Austria, Vienna General Hospital also kept careful data. Although it was a general hospital it had had lying-in wards since its establishment in 1784, and in the early years the maternal mortality rate was 12.5 per 1,000 births. This changed in 1823 when the hospital introduced the practice of routine post-mortem examinations. The maternal mortality rate quadrupled to 53 per 1,000. Ten years later the maternity service was divided into two separate clinics, with women allocated randomly to Clinic 1 or Clinic 2. The mortality rates in the two clinics were respectively 64 and 56 per 1,000 births.

In 1839 the teaching arrangements changed. Women were still allocated randomly to one or other clinic but the medical students were allocated to Clinic 1 and the midwifery students to Clinic 2. Medical students assisted at the autopsies every morning before going onto the wards, but that was not part of midwifery training. Between 1839 and 1847 the mortality rate in Clinic 1 rose to 98.4 per 1,000 while in Clinic 2 it fell slightly to 35.7.

In 1846 Ignaz Semmelweis was appointed as an assistant at the lying-in hospital. Born in Budapest in 1818, he had come to Vienna intending to study law, but he changed to medicine and qualified in 1844 (Figure 5.2). When he came to the lying-in hospital he was shocked by the mortality in Clinic 1 and determined to find the cause. In 1847 a leading forensic pathologist died after cutting his finger during an autopsy, and the findings at his post-mortem were similar to those in women who died of puerperal sepsis.

Semmelweis became convinced that the disease was transmitted by 'cadaveric particles'. He insisted students wash their hands in a disinfectant (chlorinated lime) before entering the lying-in ward. The result was that in 1848 the maternal mortality rate in Clinic 1 fell sharply to 35.7 per 1,000 – close to the rate of 30.6 in Clinic 2.

This was later seen as a milestone in maternity care but at the time very little changed. Although Semmelweis wrote to friends about his results, he did not publish them. News of his work reached London in 1849 because an Englishman, Dr Routh, was in Vienna at the time. He reported Semmelweis' work to the Royal Medical and Chirurgical Society but his published paper made no impact.

Semmelweis returned to Budapest in 1850, a significant moment in Hungary's history. In 1848, Europe's 'year of revolutions', Hungary had risen against its Hapsburg rulers but the rebellion had been put down by Austrian troops with Russian help. By the time Semmelweis returned, Hungary was under martial law and a process of 'Germanisation' had begun which lasted until 1860.

Even without this political upheaval Semmelweis had been disinclined to start writing his treatise and he did not start work on it until 1857. By then he was beginning to show signs of mental illness. The treatise, more than 500 pages long, was rambling and full of invective. It was published in 1860 and Semmelweis died in an asylum in Vienna in 1865.

For years his advocacy of handwashing was forgotten but in 1886 his reputation was restored – and enhanced – when Dr Theodore Duka, a fellow Hungarian, wrote about him in *The Lancet*. Duka blamed the Austrians for driving him out of Vienna and created a global wave of sympathy. In 1894 a meeting of leading British doctors resolved that a memorial should be erected

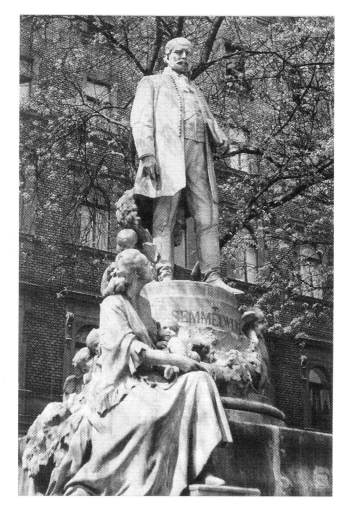

Figure 5.2 Statue of Ignaz Semmelweis (1818–65) sculpted by Alojs Stróbl in 1906. It stands in front of the Szent Rókus Hospital, Budapest.

in Budapest. A statue by Hungary's leading sculptor was unveiled in 1906 in front of an enormous crowd. Semmelweis' widow and sister were there, as were medical leaders from all over Europe, including Vienna.

Panic in England

Semmelweis had become a hero partly because of Hungarian national pride, but mainly because history showed he had been right all along. However, history took its time. Controversy about the cause of puerperal fever raged for years. In 1875 the Obstetric Society of London held a long discussion on the subject. Semmelweis' theory about 'cadaveric particles' was briefly mentioned, but not his insistence on handwashing.

The meeting had been sparked by public opinion, which seemed to be running wild. Two midwives had been charged with 'homicide by infection' after women died from puerperal infection, and one of the midwives had been put in prison. A leading article in the *Times* stated:

> *It is the invariable practice of medical men if they attend a case of this (puerperal) fever to hand over the whole of midwifery practice to other persons for at least two or three months, and it has been shown by ample experience that this course is absolutely necessary to preserve the lives of their patients.*

Dr Matthews Duncan, a leading obstetrician of the time, pointed out to the Society that 'Anything more inconsistent with the truth would be hard to find.' If the *Times* was correct, his practice and that of his colleagues would cease permanently and surgeons would also be at risk. But the law was picking on midwives, who at that time were unlicensed. Duncan added: 'I would have preferred that some *man* should have been first charged with this crime, and not a poor and comparatively defenceless woman.' The italics are his.

The meeting was attended by doctors from across the country and some spoke movingly about their anguish when an outbreak occurred in their practice. It was clear the disease was linked with erysipelas, scarlet fever and scarlatina, but there was no consensus on how to prevent it.

Home and hospital

If things were bad for doctors in practice, they were worse in hospitals. Although in Vienna General Hospital the mortality rate in Clinic 1 was now similar to rates in other lying-in hospitals, these rates were much higher than those in the community. In Queen Charlotte's Hospital, London, the mortality rate was 26 per 1,000 births – 10 times higher than that among home deliveries in the city. In Paris in the 1870s the mortality rate was 31.2 in maternity hospitals and 1.9 among charity home deliveries – a difference far too large to be explained by incomplete data collection in the community.

Lister and asepsis

This was the darkest hour before the dawn – or, rather, before two dawns. One of them broke in European laboratories and the other in British operating theatres, where Joseph Lister pioneered surgical antisepsis. The son of a Quaker, Lister had had a brilliant early career in London and Edinburgh. In 1860, at the age of 33, he was elected a Fellow of the Royal Society and was appointed Professor of Surgery in Glasgow, and in 1867 he wrote his first paper on antiseptic surgery. This involved dressings soaked in carbolic acid and the use of a continuous carbolic acid spray in the operating theatre.

Neither of these seemed appropriate to a maternity setting but, by 1882, asepsis had replaced antisepsis. Handwashing, sterilisation of instruments and drapes and general cleanliness were introduced and have been fundamental to medical practice ever since.

Lister, like Semmelweis, became a national hero. He moved as Professor of Surgery to Edinburgh and then to London but retired from practice when Agnes, his wife and lifelong supporter, died in 1893. He was created Baron Lister of Lyme Regis in 1897 and died in 1912. His memorial in Portland Place, London, was unveiled in 1924 (Figure 5.3).

Pasteur and microbiology

While Lister was transforming surgery in Britain, the science of microbiology was being born in Europe. In Paris in 1862 Louis Pasteur was awarded the Alhumbert Prize for proving the germ theory. In Berlin in 1874 Theodor Billroth first described the streptococcus and in 1879 Pasteur isolated it from cases of puerperal fever and erysipelas. The scientific revolution continued and in Berlin in the 1880s Robert Koch discovered the cause of tuberculosis. In 1905 Koch was awarded the Nobel Prize, which had been inaugurated in 1901. Pasteur and Billroth had both died in the 1890s and the Prize is not awarded posthumously.

The new science transcended national boundaries. Lister cited Pasteur in his 1867 paper and Koch attended one of Lister's lectures in London in 1881. One of Lister's many gifts was that he could see how his work and that of others fitted together. Brilliance and generosity do not always go hand in hand. In this instance there was no nationalistic or cross-channel rivalry and everyone benefitted.

A new century

The introduction of asepsis had a huge effect on hospital infection rates. The last major outbreak of puerperal fever in London's Queen Charlotte's Hospital was in 1879, when the mortality rate peaked at 40 per 1,000 births. From 1880 onwards the hospital's death rate continued to vary but was never higher than 10 per 1,000 (Figure 5.4).

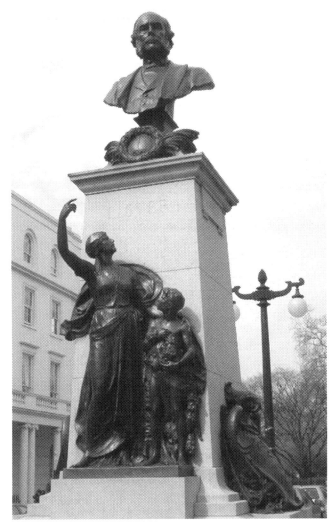

Figure 5.3 Memorial to Joseph Lister (1827–1912) in Portland Place, London, unveiled in 1924. The bust is by Thomas Brock.

National statistics mirrored the pattern of outbreaks of infection in hospitals. Across the country, from the 1840s to the 1890s, the Registrar General's figures for maternal deaths showed spikes due to puerperal sepsis as the virulence of the streptococcus waxed and waned. After 1900 these spikes were no longer seen but the baseline level did not fall. The overall maternal mortality rate remained around 4 per 1,000 births and about 40% of deaths were due to puerperal sepsis. This continued until the 1930s (Figure 5.5).

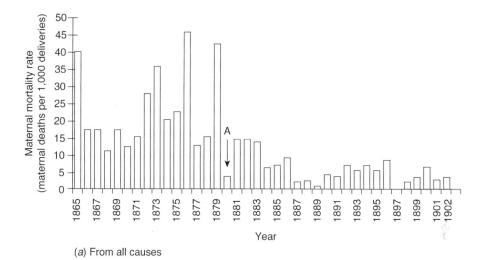

(*a*) From all causes

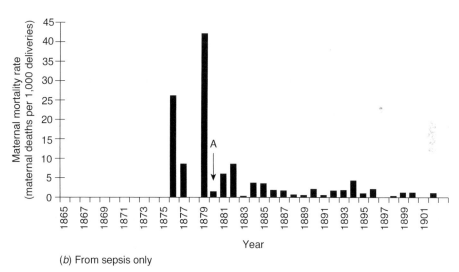

(*b*) From sepsis only

Figure 5.4 Mortality rate from sepsis at Queen Charlotte's Hospital, London, 1876–1901. Data for sepsis before 1876 are not available, but between 1865 and 1876 the hospital's overall maternal mortality rate varied between 10 and 45/1,000 births.
'A'=introduction of asepsis. From *The Tragedy of Childbed Fever* by Irvine Loudon (Oxford University Press, 2000)

Part of the trouble was that aseptic technique was difficult to maintain during birth at home or even birth in hospital. In 1933 Dr Leonard Colebrook, the director of the Research Laboratory at Queen Charlotte's Hospital, tackled the problem. Quoting the departmental report of 1932 (see Chapter 3), he wrote in the *British Medical Journal* (BMJ) that 'nearly 20% of all

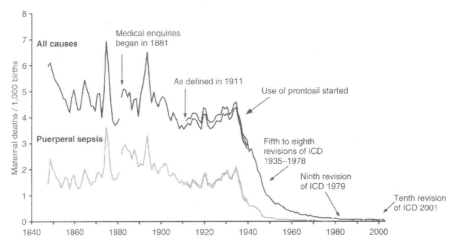

Figure 5.5 Maternal mortality rate per 1000 births, England and Wales 1840–2002.

the deaths due to child-bearing follow normal labours. If it can be proved that most of these fatal infections are due to the transfer of haemolytic streptococci to the genital tract of the woman in labour from some outside source, it means that these infections are preventable'.

Colebrook's article did indeed prove his argument. At the same time he published detailed instructions on how to improve aseptic procedures in labour. That paper, entitled 'Antisepsis in Midwifery' and also inspired by the 1932 departmental report, occupied 24 pages of the *Journal of Obstetrics and Gynaecology of the British Empire*. Colebrook's campaign might have changed practice and made a real difference to the death rate, but we shall never know because at exactly the same time a historic breakthrough was being made in Germany.

Domagk and Prontosil

The research that changed everything was done in Wuppertal by Bayer Laboratories, following a path laid out by Paul Erlich, a pupil of Robert Koch. In 1909 Erlich won the Nobel Prize for opening up the new field of chemotherapy by finding an effective treatment for syphilis. He had discovered dyes which could stain bacteria and affect their inner working, and he realised they could be developed into antibiotics. In 1929 Gerhard Domagk, a professor working on bacterial infections, was appointed to direct Bayer's research laboratory (Figures 5.6 and 5.7).

Thousands of azo dye compounds were synthesised and tested, and one of them was found to be effective against streptococci in mice. In 1935 Domagk

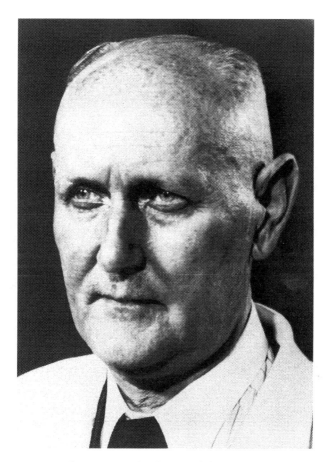

Figure 5.6 Gerhard Domagk (1895–1964)

reported an experiment in which 26 mice were infected with streptococci derived from a human infection. Fourteen were left alone and soon died but the other 12 were injected with a red dye which Domagk called prontosil. They all survived.

In London Leonard Colebrook repeated the experiment, and he reported his results in *The Lancet* in 1936. Remarkably his paper was entitled 'Treatment of Human Puerperal Infections, and of Experimental Infections in Mice, with Prontosil'. This was probably the first and certainly the only time that initial animal experiments and human trials were reported simultaneously. Colebrook felt able to do so because the mortality rate from streptococcal puerperal fever among women admitted to his specialist unit at Queen Charlotte's Hospital was between 22% and 26%. He gave prontosil to only the most seriously ill patients. Of the first 38 women treated with prontosil only 3 died. The mortality rate had been reduced to 8%.

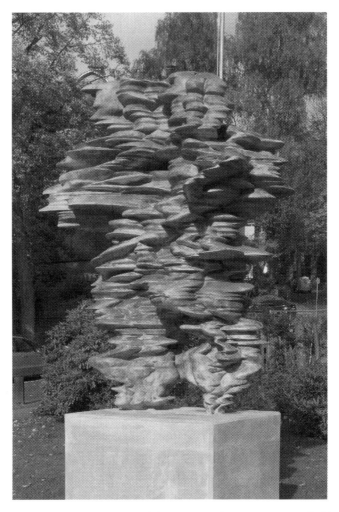

Figure 5.7 Memorial to Gerhard Domagk in Wuppertal, Germany, unveiled in 2013. The sculptor is Anthony Cragg.

The antibiotic era

Colebrook's 1936 report caused a sensation, and no wonder. This was the start of the antibiotic era. Prontosil was refined into sulphonamide and was soon followed by penicillin. Alexander Fleming had discovered this in 1928 in St Mary's Hospital, London, while working alongside Colebrook before the latter's move to Queen Charlotte's. The first attempts at purification failed, but in 1941 Howard Florey and Ernst Chain succeeded when they famously injected penicillin into an Oxford policeman. During World War II it was difficult to manufacture penicillin in quantity but, thanks to American companies, supplies increased dramatically by 1946.

In 1945 Fleming, Florey and Chain – a Scotsman, an Australian and a Jewish refugee from Germany – shared the Nobel Prize for medicine. In 1939 Domagk had been awarded the Nobel Prize but the Nazis had prevented him from accepting it. He survived the war and received the medal and the diploma (but not the cash award) in 1947. His mother did not live to see that. By then their home village was in Poland and she died in a refugee camp.

It is remarkable that the fastest-ever fall in UK maternal mortality was achieved during the chaos of World War II. In 1955 Colebrook, writing in the BMJ, summed up the transformation. Every year between 1880 and1930 there were about 2,000 maternal deaths from infection. In 1950 that figure had dropped to 21 deaths after childbirth and 64 after abortion. His paper gave credit to colleagues, including his sister Dora, who had worked alongside him in the laboratory making meticulous observations (Figure 5.8).

He believed that the fall in deaths from sepsis had not been due to drugs alone. A large number of infections, he wrote, had followed obstetric trauma due to 'unskilful or mismanaged delivery' but

> [T]he last half-century has seen great changes in obstetrics in this country. Thanks to the activities of the Royal College of Obstetricians and Gynaecologists; perhaps in some part to the report of the Ministry of Health Committee of 1928–32; but most of all, perhaps, to the conscientious effort of a host of people doing maternity work all over the world, the teaching and practice of midwifery have been greatly improved.

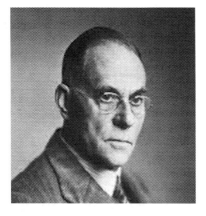

Figure 5.8 Leonard Colebrook (1883–1907).
(His sister Dora appears to have been camera-shy).

His congratulations were somewhat premature, as discussed in Chapter 4. Two years later the publication of the first CEMD Report showed that further improvement in practice was needed. Nonetheless Colebrook's comments indicate that standards had been raised from a woefully low baseline, which is why the improvement in maternal mortality during the war years was not limited to deaths from infection.

The (temporary) end of puerperal sepsis

Colebrook also warned that 'the puerperal fever hazard is *not* a thing of the past' and 'we cannot afford to let up in our aseptic and antiseptic precautions'. Deaths from infection recorded in the appendix of the CEMD Reports continued to fall, from 42 in 1952–4 to 18 in 1961–3. Most were associated with abortion and some with surgical treatment.

An increase to 28 was recorded in the Report for 1964–6, when a chapter on sepsis was introduced. Besides puerperal sepsis there were 66 deaths from sepsis following abortion and 29 following surgical treatment, making a total of 123. This fell to 88 in the next Report and 25 in 1973–5. By then the 1967 Abortion Act had taken effect and only 6 of those deaths were due to abortion, with 11 due to puerperal sepsis.

The improvement continued. In 1982–4 the chapter reported only five deaths from infection and the Report included this historic sentence: 'No deaths could be directly attributed to puerperal sepsis.' This milestone passed unnoticed. In his preface the Chief Medical Officer noted that, for the first time ever, there had been no deaths from criminal abortion, but he did not mention that the centuries-old scourge of childbed fever had come to an end.

As it turned out, however, it had only paused. Deaths from puerperal sepsis continued to appear in the CEMD Reports, in single figures apart from a peak to 11 in 1994–6. Early in the twenty-first century a new concern arose. Doctors and midwives were now unfamiliar with the early signs of infection that would have instantly rung alarm bells for their predecessors. Sepsis is often insidious in onset and can quickly become life-threatening if antibiotics are not given immediately.

In the CEMD Report for 2006–8 sepsis was once again the leading cause of direct maternal death with 26 deaths, of which 15 were due to sepsis beginning before, not after, delivery. It was essential to raise awareness. A key message of the Report was 'Be aware of sepsis – beware of sepsis', and the need for fast action was emphasised.

The message was heeded. Deaths from genital tract sepsis, having reached a 20-year high, fell to a total of 20 in the *Mothers and Babies: Reducing Risk through Audits and Confidential Enquiries across the UK (MBRRACE-UK) Report for 2009–12* (which covered a 4-year period). That Report devoted 17 pages to detailed recommendations on sepsis, including quotes from the National Institute for Health and Care Excellence and the Royal College of Obstetricians and Gynaecologists guidelines. Continuing vigilance is essential (see Chapter 14). As Leonard Colebrook predicted, the story of sepsis will never be over.

6 HAEMORRHAGE THEN AND NOW

The risk of haemorrhage stalks pregnancy. The heart pumps more than half a litre of blood every minute to the womb during the last months of pregnancy so, if uncontrolled bleeding occurs, it can rapidly become life-threatening. Haemorrhage remains the leading global cause of direct maternal deaths. It was always thus. Four centuries ago Shah Jahan built the Taj Mahal in memory of his beloved wife, Mumtaz Mahal, who died from haemorrhage after giving birth to their fourteenth child after a prolonged labour of some 30 hours.

In the first Confidential Enquiry into Maternal Deaths (CEMD) Report, covering the years 1952–4, the cause of the largest number of deaths was haemorrhage. The haemorrhages were divided into two groups according to when they occurred – before labour ('antepartum haemorrhage') or after birth ('post-partum haemorrhage'). Respectively these accounted for the deaths of 107 and 113 women which were included in the Report. Thirty-five deaths occurred from bleeding after caesarean section, but these were regarded as post-operative complications and not counted under 'haemorrhage'.

The causes of bleeding

Serious antepartum haemorrhage is usually due to one of two causes. 'Placenta praevia' is the name given to a placenta located low in the womb, below the baby. Haemorrhage is inevitable when labour begins, though bleeding may occur before that. The other cause, 'placental abruption', used to be called 'accidental haemorrhage' because it affects a normally sited placenta which strips away prematurely from the underlying womb.

Post-partum haemorrhage (PPH) usually results from failure of the uterine muscle to contract after the birth of the baby (atonic PPH). Sometimes this is due to a part or all of the placenta being retained in the womb after the birth. Post-partum haemorrhage can also be caused by tears somewhere in the genital tract after a normal birth or after the use and misuse of forceps.

The 1950s: place of birth

In the 1950s maternity care was a complex patchwork in the UK involving general practitioners (GPs), midwives and obstetricians. The places of birth were the woman's home, maternity homes overseen by GPs and hospitals with specialised facilities. A recurring theme in the early Reports was of some women giving birth in locations that were not best suited to their risk profile. Thus, one woman who had twice previously had a retained placenta was booked for a home birth, although retained placenta was well recognised then as a potentially recurring problem. She sadly died of PPH at home.

Nonetheless, haemorrhage can occur unexpectedly in women with no recognised risk features. Healthcare practitioners therefore saw the need for emergency care that could reach stricken women wherever they might be. This had to include blood transfusion.

Blood transfusion

The first-ever person-to-person blood transfusion was in fact performed by an obstetrician, James Blundell of Guy's Hospital in London, in 1818. The recipient was a woman with PPH. London was to play a central role in the development of blood transfusion in Britain. After the procedure became relatively safe (following the discovery of blood groups in 1901 and early experiments during the First World War) a blood bank was established in Camberwell, London, in 1921. It was the world's first blood donor service and donation was altruistic.

In the 1930s blood transfusion became part of the treatment of haemorrhage in pregnancy. At first this involved direct transfusion from a donor – usually one of the woman's relatives – but in 1936 Dr Malcolm Black of Glasgow recruited a panel of 200 men, most of whom lived near the maternity hospital. They were tested and registered to be called on in an emergency. A patient could be given a transfusion within half an hour of her arrival, and Black reported that a woman whose heart had stopped began breathing again after receiving 900cc of blood. Other cities organised a similar service. In Glasgow each man was entitled to receive one guinea if his blood was used, but Professor Claye of Leeds reported that 'the donors as a body have refused to accept any remuneration'.

The outbreak of the Second World War in 1939, with its threat of civilian casualties, greatly increased the need for blood transfusion, and donation centres were established across the UK. After the war, the Ministry of Health took control of blood banks and in 1946 set up the National Blood

Transfusion Service. Thus, by the 1950s when the Confidential Enquiries started, there was ready access to blood for transfusion when needed.

Ergometrine

Also available was the valuable drug ergometrine, which causes the womb muscle to contract in a sustained way. It was derived from ergot of rye – a type of fungus that grows on rye and similar plants. Since the sixteenth century it had been known that ingestion of ergot of rye could produce strong contractions of the uterus, and this was sometimes used to try to induce abortion of unwanted pregnancies.

In 1932 Chassar Moir, a Scottish obstetrician working at University College Hospital London, described powerful contractions of the uterus in women using an aqueous extract of ergot. In 1935 Moir, with Sir Henry Dale and Harold Dudley, isolated the active agent, which they named 'ergometrine'. They refused to patent its method of manufacture, which became free for anyone to use, and by the early 1940s ergometrine was well established as a drug to prevent or treat atonic PPH.

An alternative (hormonal) drug, oxytocin, was isolated in 1953 and in due course it was added to the treatment options for PPH. Later it was combined with ergometrine as 'Syntometrine', given by injection immediately after birth to reduce the risk of PPH.

Obstetric flying squads

Women who suffered major bleeding after giving birth at home or in a maternity home needed a rapid mechanism through which they could receive blood, drugs and specialised expertise. That was where the obstetric flying squads came in. H. J. Thomson founded the first obstetric flying squad in Bellshill, Lanarkshire, in 1933, and in 1935 Professor Farquhar Murray of Newcastle followed suit.

A few years later Dame Hilda Lloyd, who was to become the first female president of the Royal College of Obstetricians and Gynaecologists, described the experience of the obstetric flying squad of Birmingham, inaugurated in 1936 (Figure 6.1). Calls would come to the resident surgical officer in the hospital, who would dispatch a squad comprising an obstetrician, a midwife and a medical student (the latter there to learn and provide practical help). The aim was to reach the woman's home within half an hour of the initial call. A dedicated ambulance carried blankets, hot-water bottles, three leather bags and two sterile drums containing equipment, and two insulated boxes for blood and oxygen cylinders. It also carried lighting and, curiously, a tin of biscuits.

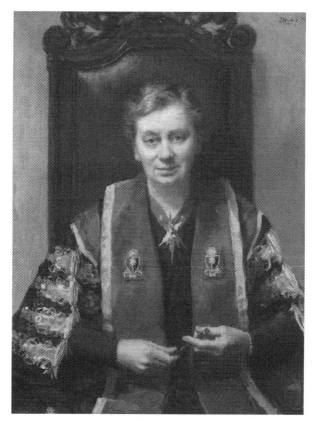

Figure 6.1 Dame Hilda Lloyd (1891–1982) was the president of the Royal College of Obstetricians and Gynaecologists (RCOG) from 1949 to 1952. Portrait by Anthony Devas. Photo courtesy of the RCOG

As flying squads evolved, it became usual for an anaesthetist to be part of the team. By the late 1980s, however, it was becoming clear that obstetric flying squads had had their day. Home births were less common and car ownership was much more widespread. Audits in Liverpool and London showed that flying squad calls had become infrequent and that few calls actually dealt with genuinely urgent problems. The conclusion was that this had now become an unnecessary and expensive practice which, in some cases, actually delayed clinical intervention. The obstetric flying squad in the UK passed into history.

The 1950s: antenatal care

The second CEMD Report, covering 1955–7, described a marked decrease in the number of deaths from haemorrhage. Particularly noticeable was the decrease in deaths associated with retained placenta. This was attributed to the increasing use of ergometrine as a treatment and a preventive measure. However, the Report's authors were concerned about the number of women who had died from haemorrhage and had never had their blood count checked during the pregnancy. Less than a third of the women had evidence of a haemoglobin check during antenatal care.

Serious haemorrhage of whatever cause obviously has greater impact on a woman who is already anaemic. (This is one reason haemorrhage remains such a serious problem in low-income countries.) The normal physiological changes of pregnancy include mild anaemia, but, in the 1950s, pathological anaemia was common among women living in poor and crowded circumstances, with unsatisfactory hygiene and nutrition, and often with a history of multiple, closely spaced previous pregnancies.

This problem was tackled by offering all women iron supplementation in the form of tablets as part of routine antenatal care. A 25-year survey of women attending antenatal clinics in Glasgow Royal Maternity Hospital recorded how practice changed. In 1951 fewer than 1% of women at the antenatal clinic were receiving iron tablets: by 1961 the figure was 50% and by 1971 it was 87%. The proportion of women who were anaemic at their first attendance in 1960 was 14.4% but in 1973 it was 1.2%. As the general health of the population improved, the need for iron supplementation was questioned.

The 1950s: antepartum haemorrhage

The 1958–60 Report highlighted the death at home of a woman who had had two vaginal examinations by her GP. She had a low-implantation placenta praevia, and the second examination provoked a catastrophic haemorrhage. In those days the diagnosis of a low-lying placenta relied on clinical grounds alone. The classical signs and symptoms were recurring small haemorrhages and an unusually high presenting part (typically the baby's head) on abdominal examination. If these were absent, the diagnosis could be very difficult indeed.

It would be many years before a report appeared of an ultrasound scan diagnosing placenta praevia. The first paper on clinical ultrasound was published by Professor Ian Donald's Glasgow team in *The Lancet* in 1958, and the first diagnosis of placenta praevia was described by Donald and Usama Abdulla in 1968. Not until 1973–5 did a CEMD Report mention ultrasound diagnosis of placenta praevia in a woman who died.

The 1960s

By 1961–3 the number of deaths from PPH had dropped dramatically to 44, from 113 in 1952–4. Only one death had occurred, in a woman transferred to hospital with a retained placenta still in place (compared to 21 in 1952–4). Removal of a retained placenta requires general anaesthesia, and the improvement was attributed to greater willingness by obstetric flying squads to induce anaesthesia in women's homes or maternity homes and extract the placenta before transfer to hospital. Inhalational anaesthesia in the woman's home was not, of course, without its own risks, as discussed in Chapter 11.

By the 1964–6 Report the number of deaths from haemorrhage had dropped still further (see Figure 6.2), but serious challenges remained. Substandard care was identified in half of the deaths. Some of the problems had been highlighted before: inappropriate booking for birth at home or in a maternity home, failure to call the obstetric flying squad until too late, and failure to check haemoglobin values during antenatal care to identify anaemia. However, this was the first Report to mention the problem of 'placenta praevia accreta'. This has remained a challenge and indeed has increased in importance until the present day.

Placenta praevia accreta

Placenta praevia, as already mentioned, is a low-lying placenta. 'Accreta' refers to an unusual degree of invasion of the placenta into the wall of the womb. This means the placenta does not separate properly after the birth of the baby and can lead to a serious and sometimes life-threatening haemorrhage. Placenta accreta can occur when the placenta is normally sited and, even then, it is very challenging to treat effectively, but placenta praevia accreta occurs when the placenta has implanted over the scar from a previous caesarean section. This makes it particularly difficult and an emergency hysterectomy may be needed to save the woman's life.

As birth by caesarean section became much more common, so too did placenta praevia accreta. The Mothers and Babies: Reducing Risk through Audits and Confidential Enquiries across the UK (MBRRACE) Confidential Enquiry, covering deaths in the UK and Ireland between 2013 and 2015, described no fewer than 9 deaths associated with placenta praevia or accreta out of a total of 22 deaths from haemorrhage. The Report reiterated the importance emphasised in previous Reports of not delaying the decision to undertake a hysterectomy when more conservative treatments were failing to keep up with blood loss in severe haemorrhage.

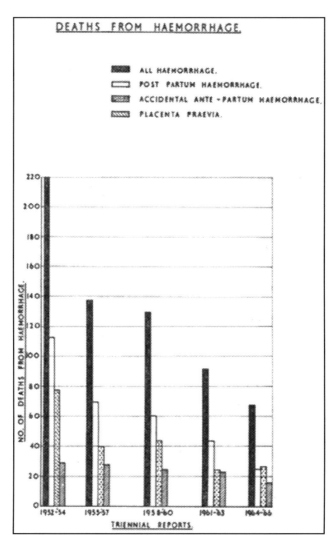

Figure 6.2 Deaths from haemorrhage, 1952–66. From the CEMD Report for 1964–6

Guidelines for emergency treatment

Dealing effectively with catastrophic haemorrhage requires the clinical team to do two things. They must tackle the root cause of the bleeding, whether this is placenta praevia or accreta, a ruptured uterus or something else altogether. At the same time, they must ensure that the woman maintains a circulating volume of physiologically useful blood. The 1979–81 CEMD Report included for the first time a written management guideline for major haemorrhage.

Guidelines have become more sophisticated since then, and new guidance is included in the recent MBRRACE report of 2020. It stresses the need for a single experienced clinician to take charge, the importance of anticipating and correcting coagulation problems and the role of a scribe to carefully document events during what is inevitably a fraught time. Simulation training and drills can be valuable in preparing clinical staff for dealing with major haemorrhage, which usually occurs suddenly and unpredictably.

Refusal of treatment

Not all women are prepared to accept transfusion of blood products. The 1973–5 Report was the first to record the death from haemorrhage of a woman who declined blood transfusion for religious reasons. In this she had the full support of her family. This and subsequent Reports led the way in moving UK maternity services to recognise this problem and to minimise risk as much as possible by planning individualised care in women such as Jehovah's Witnesses who would not accept blood products.

When a maternal death does occur in a woman with haemorrhage who does not accept blood, the central tragedy is of course the loss of that woman. However, as the 2020 MBRRACE Report highlighted, staff may also be traumatised, resulting in long-term sick leave and even in individuals leaving the profession. They too need support.

Ectopic pregnancy

Another cause of death from haemorrhage in pregnancy, recorded in a separate chapter in the CEMD Reports, is ectopic pregnancy. This is usually located in one of the fallopian tubes. The egg is actually fertilised at the far end of the tube, near the ovary, and takes days to travel to the womb, where it normally implants in the uterine wall. If implantation happens to occur before it gets there, the fallopian tube can only expand so far to accommodate the growing pregnancy before it ruptures. This can cause serious internal haemorrhage, usually in the early stages of pregnancy, requiring emergency surgery.

The first commentary on death from ectopic pregnancy in the Reports had to wait until 1964–6. Since then the Reports have highlighted recurring themes. For example, women from ethnic minority groups are over-represented among the deaths from ectopic pregnancy. It is not clear whether this is due to differences in the incidence of the disease, to difficulties in accessing appropriate clinical care or to some other issue.

Each Report documented a number of women found dead at home from ruptured ectopic pregnancies. In most cases it was unknown if the women had had symptoms or even if they knew they were pregnant. The classical symptoms of ectopic pregnancy are abdominal pain, shoulder tip pain, fainting and vaginal bleeding occurring some weeks after a missed period. However, women may have atypical symptoms, notably diarrhoea and vomiting, which are often assumed to be due to gastroenteritis, and ectopic pregnancy may not even be considered as a possibility. This can have fatal consequences.

If a woman has collapsed because of blood loss from a ruptured ectopic pregnancy, speed is of the essence. Shock from any other cause is normally treated before surgery is contemplated, but in a case of ectopic pregnancy it is important to avoid delay for resuscitation. The priority is to operate to stop the bleeding surgically.

This lesson has been learned the hard way and is an example of the need for the CEMDs' messages to be spread, not only among maternity staff, but also to teams who may encounter a pregnant woman infrequently. Their intervention can be life-saving.

7 HYPERTENSION: ENQUIRIES, TRIALS AND RECOMMENDATIONS

When the new Chicago Lying-in Hospital opened in 1931 it had an arcade with five stone plaques, each dedicated to a pioneer in maternity care (Figure 7.1). Four carried the names of long-dead European doctors (one of whom was William Smellie, mentioned in Chapter 1), but the central plaque was empty. It was waiting for the individual who would discover the cause of pre-eclampsia, then a leading cause of maternal death.

Nearly a century later the plaques are still there and the name is still missing. No one has yet found the cause of pre-eclampsia, a type of pregnancy-induced hypertension (high blood pressure). Advances in treatment, however, have greatly reduced the risk of a fatal outcome, at least in developed countries. This is not because of a breakthrough by one brilliant pioneer, but it is the result of global teamwork.

Hypertension in pregnancy

Women can have high blood pressure during pregnancy for several reasons. It might be a long-term problem that predates the pregnancy – possibly linked to another medical condition such as kidney disease. More often hypertension appears for the first time during pregnancy, usually in the second half. Of the types of hypertension occurring for the first time during pregnancy, pre-eclampsia causes most concern.

Although definitions have changed over the course of the Confidential Enquiry into Maternal Deaths' (CEMD) history of more than 50 years, pre-eclampsia is generally characterised as a condition of pregnancy in which high blood pressure and protein in the urine occur together. In early reports, the old term 'toxaemia' was used because the cause was assumed to be some kind of toxin in the bloodstream.

Pre-eclampsia may progress to eclampsia with the occurrence of epileptiform seizures. It is said that Hippocrates first described eclampsia in the fifth century BC. The name comes from the Greek word for 'a burst of light'. In the era before blood pressure could be measured or protein detected in the urine,

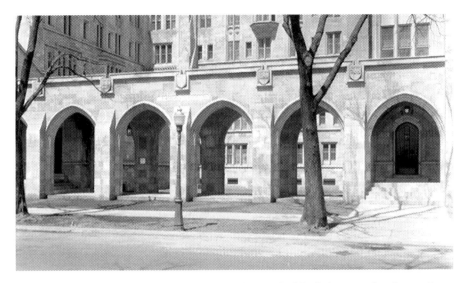

Figure 7.1 The cloister outside Chicago Lying-in Hospital, built in 1931. The plaque above the central pillar remains empty.

seizures occurred without warning. It was as if the woman had been struck by lightning.

Pre-eclampsia

The course of pre-eclampsia is highly variable. In some women the blood pressure rises slowly over days or weeks. In others it is an explosive disorder – not unlike sepsis in the speed of deterioration. The term 'fulminating pre-eclampsia' has rather gone out of fashion, but it well describes this latter pattern. Even today, eclamptic seizures sometimes occur before a documented rise in blood pressure.

Since the start of the CEMD there has been a large decrease in the number of women dying of pre-eclampsia in the UK. The first report in 1952–4 included 246 deaths. In 1976–8 there were 29, and in 2011–13 there were 6. In the words of the 2019 National Institute for Health and Care Excellence (NICE) guideline: 'There is consensus that introduction of . . . evidence-based guidelines, together with the findings from the confidential enquiry into maternal deaths, has made a pivotal contribution to this fall in maternal mortality.' This chapter will describe how the CEMD contributed to this important and welcome decline.

Globally, however, pre-eclampsia remains a very important cause of maternal deaths, being one of the five major causes along with sepsis, unsafe abortion, obstructed labour and haemorrhage. And potentially avoidable deaths still occur in the UK because further improvements are possible in the organisation and delivery of clinical care.

The role of the Confidential Enquiries

A principal benefit of the CEMD is that very rare but very important 'adverse outcomes' – that is, maternal deaths – are comprehensively scrutinised to allow lessons to be learned. Randomised controlled trials are rightly seen as the gold standard method of assessing the benefits and disadvantages of new treatments, but such trials are rarely of sufficient size to say much about very infrequent outcomes. Thus the CEMD Reports have provided complementary information to enhance the overall evidence base.

For example, CEMD Reports during the 1960s covered several fatal cases of women with rare adrenal tumours called phaeochromocytomas being mis-diagnosed with pre-eclampsia (because phaeochromocytomas also cause high blood pressure). The message of the CEMD was to consider this and other diagnoses when the pattern of high blood pressure in a pregnant woman is unusual and to investigate appropriately.

The early Reports

In the first CEMD Reports poor antenatal care was a major concern. The 1955–7 Report lamented the frequent observation of women showing signs of pre-eclampsia during antenatal care but being 'sent home to bed' and not being seen for a week or more. Those women who had not improved by then were usually – but not always – referred to hospital. The Report mentions one woman whose condition had worsened after a week. She was then sent home for 'increased rest', only to deteriorate and die.

Maternity care in the 1950s involved general practitioners, midwives and obstetricians, but they did not always work together in a well coordinated way. The timing of antenatal care visits was regimented and inflexible. This resulted in many women having an excess of antenatal care, but the converse also occurred, with women whose blood pressure had risen during antenatal care not being reviewed soon enough.

Eclampsia was a common event among the women whose deaths from pre-eclampsia were recorded in the 1950s. Eclampsia occurred in 38% in the 1952–4 CEMD Report and in 47% in the 1955–7 Report. At that time the treatment of eclampsia differed between the UK and the USA, where magnesium sulphate was used. In the UK treatment was based on sedating the woman in quiet, dark surroundings to minimise unwanted stimulation. Strong scientific evidence about the efficacy of magnesium sulphate was not to come for many years.

A better approach

The 1979–81 CEMD Report represented a real step up in analysis and advice, after a succession of dreary Reports repetitively criticising (mainly) general practitioners for poor antenatal care, but making few positive recommendations for better care of women with pre-eclampsia. The 1979–81 Report highlighted the diverse causes of death associated with eclampsia/pre-eclampsia due to fact that many organs are affected by this condition. The leading cause of death was brain haemorrhage. Other important causes were oedema (fluid retention) in the brain, failure of the liver or kidneys and heart failure.

The Report highlighted 'aspects of care in which improvement seemed particularly needed'. These included poor antenatal care (again), failure to control high blood pressure before and after birth and delay in effecting birth of the baby – which is the only cure for pre-eclampsia. The list of failings also included inadequate anticonvulsant treatment before and after birth (diazepam was the drug of choice then) and overload of intravenous fluids. In addition there were failures to anticipate complications of pre-eclampsia such as liver damage and disseminated intravascular coagulation (a life-threatening clotting disorder).

Importantly, the 1979–81 Report recommended that each UK region should have at least one team with special expertise in the care of women with severe hypertensive disease in pregnancy. These teams would provide expert advice, accept transfer of women with severe disease and set standards of care across the region. This sound advice took longer to implement than it should have, but at least this particular ball was now rolling.

Expert treatment

In the late 1980s there were concerns about the number of women with pre-eclampsia dying from breathing difficulties due to 'acute respiratory distress syndrome' (ARDS). This was attributed, at least in part, to giving excessive intravenous fluids to affected women. Pre-eclampsia can cause the blood vessels to become 'leaky', which allows the body's tissues, including lung tissue, to become waterlogged.

These observations led to the much more widespread use of written management guidelines that stressed the need for careful administration of only small amounts of intravenous fluid, under close monitoring. They also recommended obtaining advice from experts such as obstetric anaesthetists and obstetricians with special expertise in the care of women with pre-eclampsia. Today the value of using explicit guidelines and the engagement of genuine experts may seem obvious, but at the time it required a major shift in the culture of maternity units.

Protecting the brain

By 2000 deaths from ARDS had almost disappeared. The remaining challenge was intracranial haemorrhage (a type of stroke). Bleeding inside the skull or inside the brain itself had become overwhelmingly the most common way that women were dying from pre-eclampsia/eclampsia. Review of these cases in successive CEMD Reports had revealed that these women had very high blood pressures and that, in many cases, there had been inadequate attempts at using drugs to lower pressures to safer levels. The 1997–9 Report emphasised that severe hypertension is a life-threatening complication which requires rapid response and effective action. There is little to choose between the various antihypertensive drugs that are used. The important point is prompt action to rapidly initiate and maintain effective treatment.

Blood pressure measurement always gives two figures. The higher (systolic) one is the pressure at the peak of a cardiac contraction, and the lower (diastolic) figure is the sustained background pressure. Traditionally British obstetricians had focussed on the diastolic blood pressure in planning care. However, the systolic pressure – the maximum blood pressure in the artery – is likely to represent the point at which an artery in the brain would rupture, causing intracranial haemorrhage. The 2000–2 CEMD Report was very much at the vanguard of recommending that systolic pressures are taken seriously and used as an indicator of need for pressure-lowering treatment. This can be a medical emergency when these pressures are extremely high – for example, more than 200 mm Hg.

Later Reports highlighted events that can raise blood pressure to even higher levels in women already hypertensive with pre-eclampsia. Notably these include giving the drug syntometrine to prevent post-partum haemorrhage, and the effects of tracheal intubation for caesarean section under general anaesthetic, which is unusual now but sometimes is needed for speed (see Chapter 11).

The value of controlled trials

The 1991–3 Report, published in 1996, was able to highlight the landmark publication in 1995 of the Collaborative Eclampsia Trial. This was an international, multicentre, randomised controlled trial coordinated by the National Perinatal Epidemiology Unit in Oxford, UK, and published in *The Lancet*. It recruited 1,687 women with eclampsia – far more than could be studied in a single hospital or indeed a single country – and compared treatment by magnesium sulphate with the traditional British treatment by diazepam or phenytoin. The trial showed for the first time the unequivocal superiority of magnesium sulphate as an anticonvulsant for the treatment of eclampsia. The Americans had been right all along.

In the CEMD Report for 1991–3, none of the women who died from eclampsia after treatment with an anticonvulsant had received magnesium sulphate. They had received diazepam, phenytoin or chlormethiazole, or a combination of these. Treatment in the UK soon changed.

Ideally, however, eclampsia should be prevented by effective treatment of pre-eclampsia. The Oxford unit, led by Professor Lelia Duley, therefore organised another international trial – the 'MAGPIE' trial – which was conducted in 33 countries. It involved more than 10,000 women with pre-eclampsia, half of whom received magnesium sulphate and half of whom received a placebo. Published in *The Lancet* in 2002, the trial clearly showed that magnesium sulphate should be used also in the treatment of pre-eclampsia.

This was a further example of the cycle of Confidential Enquiries highlighting problems, clinical trials establishing solutions to those problems and Confidential Enquiry Reports pushing implementation of changes of practice and policy based on trial evidence.

The end result

In the past decade the number of hypertensive deaths in reported in each triennium by the UK Confidential Enquiries has been in single figures. This is an astonishing change from the 1950s, let alone the 1930s, when obstetricians – not only in Chicago – were hoping for a miracle worker. The miracle happened, but it took 70 years and it was a team effort.

8 THE STORY OF ABORTION

For 12 years from 1961 to 1972 abortion was the leading cause of maternal death in England and Wales. This was not a side effect of the 'Swinging Sixties' or the sexual revolution. It was because the number of deaths from other causes had fallen, revealing a social problem that had been killing women since the previous century.

The Confidential Enquiry into Maternal Deaths (CEMD) Reports of the time did not make recommendations about abortion. What they did do was accurately record the numbers, along with demographic information and details of the complications leading to the death. These facts, unchanging for year after year, spoke for themselves and provided a basis for political action.

The breakthrough was the Abortion Act of 1967. From a twenty-first-century perspective this seems an inevitable reform, but at the time it was highly controversial. Calls for the legalisation of abortion in the UK had begun in the 1920s and increased steadily from then on, but they were met with resistance or, worse, apathy. To understand why so many women died and how mothers' lives eventually were saved we need to begin the story further back in time.

The Victorian era

In the eighteenth century procuring an abortion was punishable by death if the attempt was made after 'quickening' (when fetal movements were felt). This law remained in effect in the nineteenth century, but, in 1803, it was extended to cover earlier stages of pregnancy. Lord Ellenborough's Act specified that 'the person so offending, their counsellors, aiders, and abetters . . . shall be liable to be fined, imprisoned, set in and upon the pillory, public or privately whipped, or transported beyond the sea for any term not exceeding fourteen years'.

In 1837 Section 58 of the Offences against the Person Act removed the distinction between pre- and post-quickening abortions and replaced the death penalty with life imprisonment for abortion at any stage of pregnancy. This applied to anyone procuring abortion, including the woman herself. In 1861 the Act was modified by adding the words 'whether she be or be not with child'. Thus the intention to procure an abortion became a crime. This law remains in force today, amended by the 1967 Abortion Act.

The law, however, was conspicuously ignored. In 1843 the forerunner of the *British Medical Journal* (BMJ) noted: 'We have heard of a French hag, living somewhere near Marylebone Lane, who enjoys no small share of fame for her success, the means which she employs consisting in the daily administration of the oils of pennyroyal and savine, with a violent cathartic at intervals of two or three days.' The BMJ listed fatalities resulting from abortifacient drugs and advised against them.

Surgical abortion (passing instruments into the uterus via the vagina) was practised by 'quack' doctors, sometimes with fatal results. After the UK Medical Register was established in 1858 surgical abortion was practised by both qualified and unqualified men. In 1885 a Mr Sprow was convicted of procuring abortion: his 'terms were £15 a year for any number of operations required to keep a married woman free from children'.

The exact prevalence of abortion in the nineteenth century is not known, but it was certainly common. After the Industrial Revolution the population of England increased fivefold and families in the rapidly expanding cities lived in festering slums. Mrs Gaskell, wife of a Unitarian minister, shocked her readers with the realities of life for poor women in Manchester. She described the seduction, prostitution and suicide of her heroines but never mentioned abortion.

Nonetheless she knew about it. When her friend the novelist Charlotte Bronte died in early pregnancy from pregnancy vomiting (a condition which then could be cured only by abortion) Mrs Gaskell wrote in a letter: 'How I wish I had known! I do fancy that if I had come, I could have induced her, – even though they had all felt angry with me at first, – to do what was so absolutely necessary, for her very life. Poor poor creature!'

In 1869 the BMJ described the frequency of abortion in the USA, where abortifacients were openly advertised, and gave convincing evidence that abortions were easily obtained in England. Infanticide was also common, with 'mill-ponds, in the neighbourhood of factories, that have been made the receptacles for many a new born child'. At that time there was no legal requirement to register a stillbirth.

In 1873 the British Medical Association (BMA) lobbied for such registration, asserting that 'children killed during birth and after birth are doubtless buried as still-born'. It cited a case 'at Plymouth, where one midwife appeared at a cemetery so constantly with the bodies of children for burial as still-born, that suspicion was excited'.

In 1896 a midwife was sentenced to death for procuring an abortion which ended with the death of the woman. The BMA stated that 'it is now customary to teach pupil midwives … the symptoms and treatment of abortion and miscarriage … this practice is unsound and directly leads to the practice of Criminal Abortion'. The BMA opposed the registration and of midwives, ostensibly for this reason, but the Midwives Act was finally passed in 1902. Stillbirth registration, however, was not introduced in England and Wales until 1927.

Opinion starts to shift

At the beginning of the twentieth century the law continued to turn a blind eye to abortion by qualified medical practitioners. Requests were commonplace. Letters to the BMJ claimed, 'The crime is now looked on in fashionable circles as no crime at all, and women are not a bit ashamed of asking a physician to commit the crime of foeticide', and that 'the diminishing birth-rate is due in a very large measure to the unblushing, wholesale and systematic practice of inducing abortion'.

In 1921, however, the royal gynaecologist stated that in 35 years of private practice he had carried out only 57 abortions, all of them for life-threatening indications such as placenta praevia, breast cancer and 'mental aberration' leading to intractable vomiting (the condition which had carried off Charlotte Bronte). He added: 'I know of no more difficult vaginal operation than the removal of a 16–20 weeks' pregnancy by means of ovum forceps after rapid dilatation.' It was not a procedure for amateurs.

Nevertheless criminal abortion flourished. In 1920 *The Lancet* noted 'the increase of the practice of abortion during the circumstances produced by the war, the public conscience being dead to it'. In Germany the ratio of abortions to births reached one to two in Hamburg and more than four to five in Berlin. In England a judge, sentencing an abortionist to 10 years' penal servitude for manslaughter, regretted that the charge had not been murder, which would have meant a death sentence. He commented: 'A country which permits its population to be dealt with in this way is bound to decay. Those who have as many enemies as the British Empire must for their own safety have plenty of children to meet those enemies in the gate.'

During the 1920s opinion began to shift. Although it was widely accepted that a doctor acting in good faith would not be prosecuted, *The Lancet* pointed out in 1927 that the act prohibiting abortion was 90 years old and suggested that 'if it were re-enacted again today an express proviso would be inserted to exempt from criminal liability the fully qualified practitioner who terminates a pregnancy for the bona fide purpose of preserving the mother from special danger to life or health'. The final two words are important.

The Infant Life (Preservation) Act 1929

In 1929 an act was quietly passed to remedy a perceived legal anomaly. During the trial of someone alleged to have murdered a child during its birth, a judge had held that it was illegal to murder a child before or after birth, but not during the process of birth itself. The Infant Life (Preservation) Act of 1929 introduced the offence of 'child destruction' – causing the death of an unborn child capable of being born alive 'before it has an existence independent of its mother'.

The intention was to close a legal loophole, but the Act went further by stating that no offence was committed if the person caused the child's death in good faith for the sole purpose of preserving the life of the mother. Putting these words into law carried the implication that abortion for any indication other than saving the mother's life was now illegal, putting doctors in greater jeopardy than they had been in before.

Pressure builds: the 1930s

In 1932 *The Lancet* again asked, 'Should abortion be legalised?' At a meeting of the Medico-Legal Society of London 'legal opinion was universally in favour of a modification of the law in this country or even of legalisation of abortion, while with few exceptions the medical members present supported the present position'. Citing the 'satisfactory statistics ... accumulated during ten years' experience of legalised abortion in modern Russia', *The Lancet* called for 'new legislation appropriate to the outlook and habits of our times'.

The 'present position' was that abortion was left to the discretion of doctors, most of whom preferred not to talk about it openly. However, one professor of midwifery wrote in the BMJ: 'The man in the street knows perfectly well that on the Continent he can arrange for an undesired pregnancy to be terminated, and I have heard it stated that if he knows his way about it he need not trouble to leave this country; the necessary medical indication will be found.' Regretting that the 1929 Act had been so restrictive, he suggested a list of indications including previous caesarean section, a family of 10 or more, or 'going abroad to join her husband where medical assistance was not easily obtainable'.

An abortion by a qualified private practitioner was beyond the means of most women, and evidence of the ill effects of the 'present position' began to accumulate. The League of Nations reported that 'as a cause of maternal deaths abortion has become more important than delivery at term'. In Germany 8,000 women died from abortion every year. In London a leading obstetrician, Francis J. Browne, a professor at the University of London, estimated that abortion accounted for 25% of maternal mortality in England.

The methods used for illegal abortion had not changed since Victorian times. In a survey of 23 criminal abortions in Glasgow, 14 resulted from drugs, including ergot, and 9 from the use of instruments including a knitting needle, a crochet hook and a catheter. A survey in Liverpool classified methods as (1) general violence, including rolling downstairs, (2) internal administration of drugs (which had to be given in large enough doses to endanger the life of the woman), (3) direct violence, including uterine sounds and umbrella ribs, and (4) injection of fluids such as soap solutions. In fatal cases death was either quick due to shock or air embolism, or a lingering process due to sepsis.

In 1936 *The Lancet* repeated its call for a change in the law. It doubted whether compulsory notification of abortion was practicable but suggested that two doctors should be involved in the decision and added, 'Feminine opinion, never so well organised or so articulate as today, will no doubt be heard.'

Women had indeed found their voice. In 1936 the Abortion Law Reform Association (ALRA) was founded by a small group already active in promoting information about contraception for working-class women. At first it had 35 members but in 1939 it had almost 400. In the same year a deputation from the National Council of Women led by Lady Astor, MP, urged the government to investigate the role of criminal abortion in maternal mortality.

Government action followed. In 1937 a major report by the Ministry of Health focussed on areas with the highest maternal mortality rates (see Chapter 2). The Report noted 'frequent assertions … that women became debilitated … as a result of the repeated and prolonged use of aperients and other drugs taken with the object of terminating pregnancy', and that 'it seems evident that the practice of artificially induced abortion is increasing, is more prevalent in some districts than in others, and is not restricted to any one social class'. It concluded that 14% of all puerperal deaths were due to abortion, 'excluding deaths from abortion classed as criminal'. (This exclusion suggests that Browne's estimate was not far off the mark.)

The Home Secretary and the Minister of Health immediately set up an inter-departmental committee 'to inquire into the prevalence of abortion, and the law relating thereto, and to consider what steps can be taken by more effective enforcement of the law'. It was chaired by Norman Birkett (a leading lawyer and a former Methodist lay preacher, later Lord Birkett) and included Mrs Stanley Baldwin (the prime minister's wife) and Mrs Dorothy Thurtle (a member of the ALRA). It reported in 1939. It strongly opposed any broad relaxation of the law but recommended that the law should make it 'unmistakeably clear that a medical practitioner is acting legally, when in good faith he procures the abortion [of a pregnancy] likely to endanger the woman's life or seriously impair her health'.

Mrs Thurtle submitted a minority report which would allow abortion after four pregnancies, after rape or incest and in mental and physical defectives. Birkett had some sympathy with her view and wrote a foreword for her book *Abortion Right or Wrong*, published in 1940. Later another ALRA founding member, Alice Jenkins, published a book, *Law for the Rich*, in which she described how abortion was easily available to well-off people with the right contacts, and asked, 'Could this help not be extended to poverty-stricken women in the lower income groups?'

The Bourne Case

In 1938 Aleck Bourne, a gynaecologist at St Mary's Hospital, London, decided to put the legal position of doctors to the test (Figure 8.1). A 14-year-old girl pregnant after violent rape by a group of soldiers had been referred to him by Dr Joan Malleson, another founding member of the ALRA. Bourne (who was also a member of the ALRA) carried out an abortion and informed the police. His trial attracted much media attention. Witnesses in his support included the royal gynaecologist, Mr (later Sir) William Gilliatt, and the king's physician, Lord Horder. The judge summed up sympathetically (pointing out that the girl

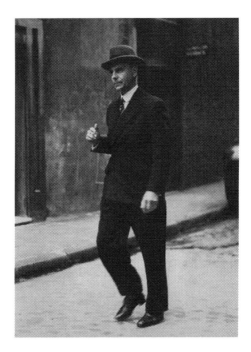

Figure 8.1 Aleck Bourne leaving Marylebone Police Court during his trial, 1st July 1938.

was 'not of the prostitute class but an ordinary decent girl') and the jury took only 40 minutes to return a verdict of not guilty.

Bourne, the son of a Wesleyan minister, wanted only to clarify the legal position of a doctor carrying out an abortion in good faith and was dismayed when he was swamped with requests after the trial. His entry in the *Dictionary of National Biography* comments that 'The case may well have sown the seeds of further relaxation of the law and the controversy it generated may have cost Bourne his chance of high office in the Royal College of Obstetricians and Gynaecologists.' Further calls for a change in the law followed, but the issue disappeared when war broke out in 1939.

The 1950s

During the war maternal mortality fell dramatically (see Chapter 5) but, as far as abortion was concerned, nothing changed, even when the National Health Service (NHS) was established in 1948. During post-war reconstruction women's issues were not a priority, and no government dared touch the controversial subject of abortion. The Bourne case may actually have been counterproductive: Home Secretary Richard Austen Butler cited it as the reason further parliamentary action was not needed.

Surveys of illegal practice continued to appear in the BMJ. In 1950 a review of 2,665 abortions in a working-class suburb of London reported that most abortions were self-induced, either medicinally or with douching, usually with soapy water. 'A curious specialty of the district was a tablespoon of powdered ergot taken in a wineglassful of hot port.' The report added that 'midwives and others acting as professional abortionists' usually preferred a douche, but some 'stirred up' the uterine contents with a long sound. All but one of the six deaths covered in the review followed douching. One patient had injected fluid from a syringe with such force she had ruptured her uterus.

In 1951 a report to the Medico-Legal Society described a typical abortion service. It was organised around a dance hall: clients were directed to the railway station, where they were met by a car and given further instructions. 'The gentleman who carried out the abortions charged anything from 20 to 100 guineas', and his method was evidently surgical: of the 89 deaths in this report the commonest cause was peritonitis. Many abortionists, however, provided prophylactic sulphonamides, reducing the number of deaths due to infection and increasing the proportion due to haemorrhage and air embolism. The fees varied according to the woman's means – as they did in the USA, where in 1960 Alfred Kinsey reported that the financial cost of abortion 'appears to vary directly with the age of the patient but is least for hospital staff'.

The Confidential Enquiries

The first Report of the CEMD, covering the years 1952–4, appeared in 1957. It had a short chapter on abortion, which was the third commonest cause of maternal death after hypertensive disease and haemorrhage. Two-thirds of abortion deaths were classified as 'avoidable' because they had been illegally procured. The Report concluded: 'It has only been possible to indicate some features of a social problem that is mainly outside the scope of this Enquiry.'

Of the 153 deaths, 108 followed abortions known to have been procured, in 58 cases, by the woman herself. The remaining cases were classed as 'uncertain'. Figure 8.2 shows the effect of social class as described at the time: only 2 cases came from the class which could afford private medical care. Noting that more than 80% of the deaths were of married women, the Report allowed its impassive mask to slip by commenting that most were 'mothers of families', and 21'were noted to be living under poor conditions and the struggle to keep a home together must have been severe'.

The next two Reports painted a similar picture, and the lack of change became increasingly conspicuous as deaths from other causes fell dramatically. The Report for 1961–3 recorded: 'Procured abortion, a special largely social problem, is now the commonest cause of avoidable maternal death.' The 139 deaths from abortion showed only a slight fall since the first Report, while both of the two previous leading causes, toxaemia and haemorrhage, had fallen by around 60%.

The Report for 1964–6 included 133 deaths, of which 74% were known to have followed illegal interference, and for the first time mentioned ethnicity:

Table XI

Circumstances			Single	Married
Well to do	...	...	1	1
Comfortable	...	...	12	42
Poor	...	...	3	20
Destitute	...	...	—	1
Not noted	...	...	6	21
			22	85

Figure 8.2 Number of deaths by social class and marital status, CEMD Report for 1952–4

24 of the women were described as 'coloured'. It included a detailed description of the geographical distribution: more than 50% of the deaths occurred in the four metropolitan regions.

The 1967 Abortion Act

Between 1950 and 1967 four attempts were made to change the law. Bills were presented in 1952, 1961, 1965 and 1966 – all drafted by Glanville Williams, a leading jurist who was a professor at University College London and later at Cambridge University. A Welshman raised in a pious Congregationalist family, Williams became the chairman of the ALRA in 1962.

Normally bills are introduced by the government, but Parliament has a system of 'Private Members' Bills' introduced by Members of Parliament (MPs) whose names are drawn out of a ballot. In 1952 Joseph Reeves was unexpectedly successful and decided to introduce a bill legalising abortion. No draft had been prepared, but Alice Jenkins contacted Glanville Williams, who swiftly produced one. It was attacked by Cardinal Griffin, a former archbishop of Westminster, and only five minutes were allowed for debate on a Friday afternoon in 1953.

Further attempts also failed through lack of parliamentary time but in 1967 David Steel was better prepared. Steel, the son of a Church of Scotland minister, had been elected to Parliament in 1965 at the age of 26 (Figure 8.3). He had been influenced by Professor Dugald Baird of Aberdeen (Figure 8.5), who had studied the effect of social conditions on women's health, and by Vera Houghton (Figure 8.4), a member of the ALRA since 1951 and its chair since

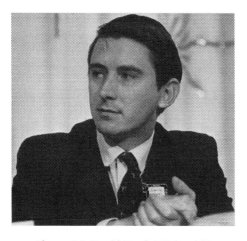

Figure 8.3 David Steel, MP, in 1967

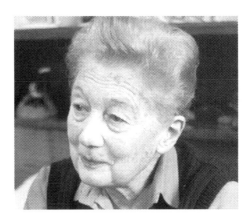

Figure 8.4 Vera Houghton (Lady Sowerby) in 1988

1963. When Steel's name happened to be drawn, he chose to reintroduce the abortion bill.

As a member of the tiny Liberal Party, Steel had to enlist the help of Peter Jackson and Sir George Sinclair (Labour and Conservative MPs respectively) to persuade members to give up their Fridays for a succession of free votes. These 'unofficial whips' were supported by Alastair Service, the ALRA's parliamentary officer, whom Steel later called 'a one-man walking whip's office'.

The Labour government was supportive and appointed a committee to advise on the bill. It was chaired by Sir John Peel, the royal gynaecologist, the president of the Royal College of Obstetricians and Gynaecologists (RCOG) and the son of a Methodist minister. Driven by the need to reduce maternal mortality, he persuaded the RCOG to support the bill. As his obituary put it when he died aged 100: 'The college council contained a number of distinguished gynaecologists who were deeply unhappy with the proposed new law. The balanced college view that emerged owed much to John's skilful handing of the council, where arguments were often very strong and passions high.'

The same applied in the House of Commons, but the bill passed and received royal assent on 27 October 1967. The fact that it did so was the result of Steel's political skill. Opponents of abortion wanted none of it, and the ALRA wanted abortion to be free of any legal constraints. The latter were disappointed by the act's requirement for a form with the signatures of two doctors and the need for the Department of Health to be notified of all abortions. These compromises had been necessary, however, to get the bill through.

After 1967

The Abortion Act divided medical opinion, and deep divisions in the profession remained for many years. Aleck Bourne opposed the Abortion Act and, in 1966, he became a founding member of the Society for the Protection of the Unborn Child. All he had wanted was to free doctors from the threat of police action when they terminated a pregnancy after careful consideration. Sir John Peel had reservations about the subsequent working of the Abortion Act and became a patron of the organisation Doctors Who Respect Human Life.

Hugh McLaren, a member of the RCOG Council under Peel's presidency, remained a leading opponent of the Abortion Act. He was a professor of obstetrics and gynaecology in Birmingham, and it was clear NHS abortions would never become available there until he retired. As soon as the Abortion Act was passed its supporters set up the Birmingham Pregnancy Advisory Service as a charity. It later became the British Pregnancy Advisory Service and continues to this day.

In other cities small private abortion clinics were set up for the same reason, and abortion moved from the back streets to the leafy suburbs, where women still had to pay the clinics' fees. Across the country the opinions of influential local obstetricians were paramount. In Aberdeen Professor Baird had implemented a liberal policy (with the support of the local police) long before the law changed, but in Glasgow Professor Ian Donald (the pioneer of ultrasound) was an outspoken opponent of the Abortion Act (Figure 8.6).

The availability of abortion through the NHS remained patchy for many years. In 1992 the proportion of abortions carried out by the NHS was 84% in Northumberland and 36% in Yorkshire. It was calculated that, over the previous 25 years, around £10 million had been paid in Yorkshire by 'women in trouble, and those who could least afford it'. If they had lived a few miles to the north, abortion would have been free.

The effect on maternal mortality

Despite these inequalities the Abortion Act eventually ended death from illegal abortion, but it took 15 years to do so. Abortion remained the leading cause of maternal death in 1967–9, when 55% of the 117 deaths were due to sepsis and 34% were of 'coloured women', and in 1970–2, when one-third of the 81 deaths were of 'women born in the New Commonwealth'. However, deaths after 'spontaneous' abortion disappeared almost completely, confirming that all along they had been due to illegal intervention.

In the early years after the Act deaths following legal abortion increased (Figure 8.7). In 1970–2 these totalled 37, of which 25 followed second-trimester

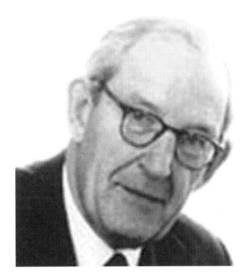

Figure 8.5 Sir Dugald Baird (1899–1986)

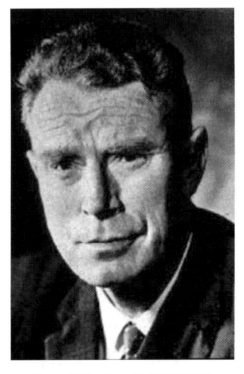

Figure 8.6 Ian Donald CBE (1910–87)

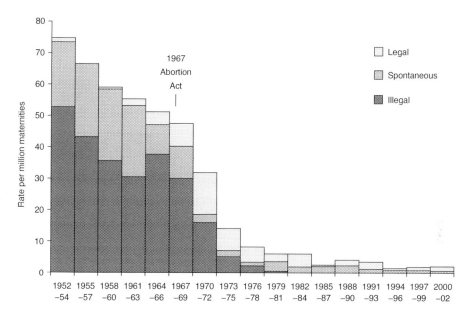

Figure 8.7 Rates of maternal death from legal, spontaneous and illegal abortions, 1952–2002

abortions – a difficult operation, as the royal gynaecologist had pointed out in 1921, requiring skill which may not have been available in small private clinics. The use of prostaglandins for safe induction of mid-trimester abortions was first described in 1971, and this later became a possible alternative to the technically difficult 'dilatation and evacuation' or other risky procedures.

At last in 1982–4 there were no deaths from illegal abortion (though one death after 'spontaneous abortion' was suspicious). The total number of deaths after abortion in that triennium was 11, and the Report made recommendations about emergency procedures in abortion clinics. This was the last Report with a separate chapter on deaths after abortion. From 1985–7 onwards they were included under 'Early pregnancy deaths' and deaths after abortion or miscarriage remained in single figures.

Prevalence of abortion

After the Abortion Act came into force in 1968 all abortions had to be reported to the Department of Health, and official statistics became available for the first time. Within five years the annual total of legal abortions to women resident in Britain had risen above 120,000 (Figure 8.8). In 1966 estimates of annual abortion numbers varied from 87,000 to 100,000 – the latter being the figure published in *Hansard*. Such estimates usually turned out to be low, so it seems likely that most, if not all, of the rapid post-1967 increase was due to the reporting of abortions which would previously have been illegal.

The other sea change in women's reproductive health during the 1960s was that effective methods of contraception became more widely available. Disappointingly, this did not lead to a reduction in the number of abortions. Campaigners in the 1930s had said that abortion and contraception went hand in hand and it was unrealistic to expect one to replace the other. As Figure 8.8 shows, time has proved them right.

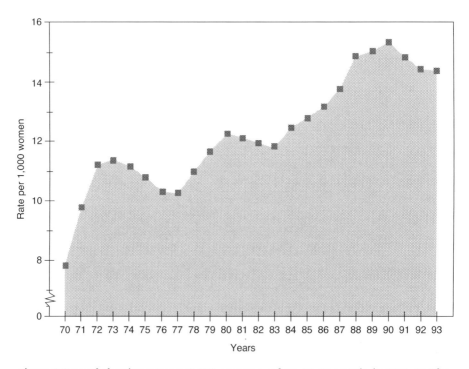

Figure 8.8 Legal abortion rate per 1,000 women aged 15–44, Great Britain 1970–93. The peak in 1973 represents a total of just over 120,000 abortions. Graph from the CEMD Report for 1991–3

Conclusion

The issue of abortion remains contentious and is discussed mainly in terms of gender politics and religion. A century ago it was a class issue. Doctors believed the decision should be theirs alone and fought to retain that right. While the debate continued, women died. Eventually the death toll forced a consensus that action was needed, but parliamentary action required diplomacy and political skill. Medicine and politics often work together, but, in this story, more than any other featured in this book, politics played the bigger role in saving women's lives.

9 CHALLENGING TRADITION: THE STORY OF EMBOLISM

In December 1947 the *British Medical Journal* (BMJ) published a paper entitled 'The Dangers of Going to Bed'. It was written by a London physician, Richard Asher (father of the actress Jane). He became famous within medicine for challenging tradition and many of his papers, including that one, are now seen as classics. The tradition of bed rest goes back a long way. For centuries doctors and patients saw it a cure for all ills, especially after childbirth. Asher, however, gave a long list of its complications, among which was the lethal condition thromboembolism.

Thrombosis is the formation of blood clots within arteries or veins. Embolism occurs when a clot breaks off and lodges elsewhere. During pregnancy blood is more liable to clot and the risk is also increased by venous stasis – slowing of blood flow in the legs due to bed rest or to the uterus pressing on the pelvic veins. Clots which form in these veins can break away, travel to the lungs and block the pulmonary (lung) circulation with fatal results.

For many years medical students were taught that the clinical picture of pulmonary embolism (PE) is of a patient who sits up in bed, calls for a bedpan and drops dead. Death was sudden and unpredictable – an 'Act of God' – and it seemed that nothing could be done to prevent it. Pulmonary embolism was the fourth commonest cause of death in the Confidential Enquiry into Maternal Deaths (CEMD) Report for 1952–4 but was summarised in only two pages. It had caused 138 deaths, 93.5% of them classed as 'unavoidable'. With hindsight most of these deaths can be blamed on the tradition of prolonged bed rest after birth.

Bed rest after delivery

'Lying-in' after childbirth is mentioned in manuscripts from the fifteenth century, and its long tradition is entirely understandable. Before the introduction of caesarean section in the nineteenth century a painful labour could last for days, birth was often traumatic and bleeding could be life-threatening. Women needed time in bed to recover. In 1752 a leading obstetrician, William

Smellie, described the tender care to be given to women 'from the time of their delivery to the end of the month'.

Even then, however, some obstetricians recognised the risks. In 1773 Charles White of Manchester gave a lurid description of how women, both rich and poor, were forced to lie for days wrapped up tightly in bed. 'The sooner she gets out of bed the better; this should not be deferred beyond the second or third day at the furthest.'

In the nineteenth century the puerperium (the recovery period after child-birth) was carefully studied. It takes about two months for the uterus to return to its normal size and position, and some doctors thought that getting out of bed too early could disturb this process or even cause prolapse. Damage to the pelvic muscles from vaginal delivery was a concern then – as it is today – and prolonged bed rest was believed to promote their healing.

Ten to 14 days in bed became the norm. In 1900 the Glasgow Obstetrical and Gynaecological Society was told, 'Rising before the fourteenth day, when the process of healing is well advanced, is detrimental. After this period, continued rest will be harmful ... The examination of the uterus by palpation gives a good guide as to when it is safe for the rigour of the confinement to be relaxed.' The word 'confinement', with its implication of immobility, remained in common use until the 1950s.

Early ambulation

By the 1930s, however, change was in the air. In 1923 Dr Benge Atlee, at the young age of 33, was appointed a new professor at Dalhousie University in Nova Scotia. He was ahead of his time in many ways. In 1935 he wrote: 'I propose to call the traditional handling of the puerperium into question. I do so with considerable diffidence, since the two classical obstetrical textbooks of this continent are on the side of tradition.'

At that time the 'standard textbook' was regarded as the ultimate medical authority. In America *Williams' Obstetrics*, written by John Whittridge Williams of Baltimore, had appeared in 1903. (Today it is in its twenty-fifth edition, written by multiple authors.) Joseph B. De Lee of Chicago published *The Principles and Practice of Obstetrics* in 1913 and it lasted for 13 editions. In 1935 both authors, described later as 'the titans of 20th century obstetrics', were advising two weeks' bed rest after normal delivery.

Atlee, by contrast, encouraged women to get out of bed on the third day. In his 1935 paper he reported that they suffered no harmful effects and indeed reacted with enthusiasm. Later, in 1953, he wrote that among 2,632 cases followed for up to 22 years, 'we have no evidence that early ambulation increases the incidence of embolism but rather the contrary'. Indeed there had been only one 'mild, non-fatal' case. His 1953 report appeared in what is now the *British Journal of Obstetrics and Gynaecology*. In it, Atlee commented that Dr De Lee had criticised his 1935 paper but his textbook had changed its advice after his death.

By the early 1950s studies in the USA had shown the safety of ambulation on day one after delivery. In Britain the lesson was learned in other ways. In 1955 Dr K. D. Salzmann recalled that, in a general practice obstetric unit near London, 'whenever the sirens sounded during the war all mothers who had reached the second day of the puerperium walked unassisted downstairs to shelter in the basement. They appeared to benefit, not suffer, from this early ambulation.'

That unit changed its routine to allow women out of bed on day three and Dr Salzmann reported in the BMJ that 'well over 1000 have tried and applauded the new regime'. He noted that Atlee had disproved the fears about prolapse, but even so, 'better far be alive with a prolapse than dead with a pulmonary embolism. There is many a good woman now lying in her grave because she was kept too long lying in her bed after an operation or confinement.'

Nevertheless most British obstetricians remained cautious. In 1960 the ninth edition of F.J. Browne's standard textbook, *Antenatal and Postnatal Care*, advised mobility 'by means of suitable exercises and early ambulation' but also recommended adequate rest. It stated that 'every patient should be examined at the end of the lying-in period, usually, therefore eight to ten days after delivery'.

The CEMD gets involved

The early CEMD Reports were reluctant to express an opinion about ambulation. Both the 1955-7 and 1958-60 Reports concluded: 'The records do not provide enough information to determine the relationship between ambulation and the occurrence of the embolism, but it is clear that the majority were walking about.' Later it was discovered that thrombosis can begin silently while a woman is in bed. It may be days or weeks before embolism follows. In the 1950s, however, techniques for diagnosing silent thrombosis in leg veins were not available. It would take 20 years for tests such as Doppler ultrasound and radioactive fibrinogen to arrive, and it would be unfair to blame the early CEMD assessors for drawing the wrong conclusion from the fact that most of the women who died 'were walking about'.

What they did do, though, right from the start, was to divide deaths from embolism into three groups: deaths during pregnancy, after vaginal delivery and after caesarean section. Over the next decade clear differences emerged among the groups. Deaths during pregnancy and after caesarean section hardly changed but deaths after vaginal delivery fell from 114 in 1955–7 to 66 in 1961–3.

The CEMD tried to gather more data but information was hard to find, particularly about ambulation. The CEMD introduced a special form for deaths from PE and the 1961–3 Report commented, 'it is hoped that [it] will be completed in all cases. In this series only thirteen forms were returned'. In 1964–6 the form was completed in 76 of the 95 cases and the chapter, now eight pages long, identified risk factors such as age, obesity, traumatic delivery and caesarean section.

It also discussed the possibility that warning symptoms may have been ignored and raised the question of treatment by anticoagulants. This was a controversial issue. Massive haemorrhage was the childbirth complication obstetricians feared most, and they were understandably reluctant to give women anti-clotting drugs.

The CEMD focussed increasingly on identifying women at risk. In the 1973–5 Report a section on possible causative factors discussed not only the ones already identified but also ABO blood groups, sickle cell disease and the suppression of lactation by oestrogens. Oestrogens, introduced for this purpose in the 1940s, were still being used although they had been shown to be ineffective. Meanwhile deaths continued to fall.

The dramatic reduction is shown in Figure 9.1. Deaths after vaginal delivery (identified by the white bars) fell to 15 in 1973–5 and by the end of decade were in single figures. It seems obvious now that the main reason for this spectacular improvement was early ambulation, but it is surprisingly difficult to find hard data in the medical journals of the time. Some information, however, comes from a non-medical source.

Women's voices

By the 1980s in Britain the time-honoured tradition of 'doctor knows best' was being challenged. In particular, the specialty of obstetrics and gynaecology was experiencing a cold blast of consumerism, and the spotlight fell on maternity services. In 1981 the BBC television programme *That's Life* asked viewers, 'What is it like to have a baby in Britain today?' It received nearly 10,000 letters and sent out questionnaires to everyone who had written. A book based on the 6,000 replies, *The British Way of Birth*, was published in 1982 (Figure 9.2).

The British Way of Birth included a section about the postnatal ward. Respondents reported good and bad experiences there, but a consistent picture

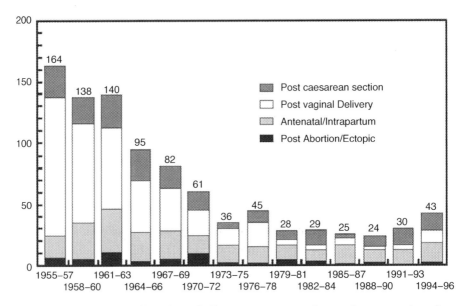

Figure 9.1 Deaths from thromboembolism, 1955–96. Note the numbers occurring after normal birth.

emerged of how long women spent in hospital. A quarter had stayed for 48 hours or less. For under a third the stay was more than six days, mostly after caesarean section or a first birth, or because of a medical problem. The book's editors commented that 'the stay in hospital had reduced steadily during the last decade'.

This change accelerated during the 1980s. Postnatal units reduced in size – a trend that has continued to the present day. Between 1987 and 2020 the number of maternity beds in English hospitals halved from 15,932 to 7,663. It is difficult to say whether this change was due to consumerism, cost-saving or a combination of the two, but by then these were the main driving forces in maternity care, rather than the need to save women's lives.

Caesarean Section

Once deaths after vaginal birth had fallen, attention turned to caesarean section. There were only 4 deaths after vaginal birth in 1991–3 but deaths after caesarean section increased to 13. This was due to a dramatic rise in Britain's caesarean section rate.

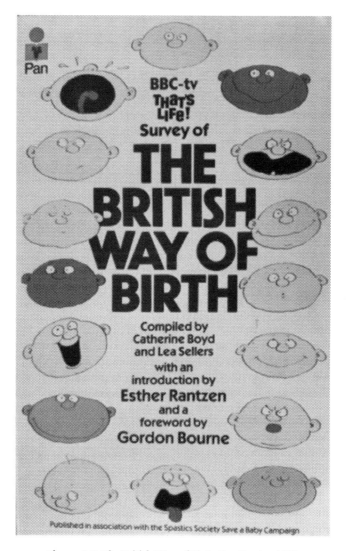

Figure 9.2 *The British Way of Birth*, Pan Books, 1982

In the 1950s only about 3% of births had been by caesarean section. Over the years the proportion climbed steadily to 10% in the early 1980s and 19% in 1999. During those five decades caesarean section had become much safer and the risk to each individual woman had diminished. Nevertheless, the sixfold increase in the number of operations, coupled with changes in other risk factors, led to a rise in the total number of deaths from PE.

Attempts to reduce the caesarean section rate were unsuccessful. Nobody wanted to go back to the days of difficult vaginal delivery (see Chapter 4), and neither doctors nor women were willing to risk the baby's life when signs of fetal distress (possible lack of oxygen) developed during labour. The World Health Organization arbitrarily set a limit of 15% on the global caesarean section rate, but in country after country the rate increased beyond that. In Britain it continued to rise to 25% and beyond.

Rather than trying to turn back the clock, doctors had to tackle the potential complications of caesarean section one by one in order to minimise the overall risk. Thromboembolism was high on the list.

Hysterectomy

Gynaecology was facing a similar problem. Surveys in the 1980s found that more than 20% of women felt that their periods were seriously interfering with their lives, and hysterectomy rates rose because less drastic options for eliminating menstruation were not yet available. In 1995 more than 20% of British women over the age of 50 had had a hysterectomy. Laparoscopic ('keyhole') surgery was still in its infancy and only one-third of those operations were carried out by the vaginal route, which is safer but technically more difficult than operating via the abdomen. Of the 93,000 women who underwent hysterectomy in 1995, two-thirds had a major abdominal operation followed by six or more days in bed in hospital. Although pregnancy was not a risk factor, the combination of pelvic surgery and immobility put them at risk of thromboembolism.

In the 1980s surgeons and anaesthetists established a national enquiry, modelled on the CEMD, into surgical mortality. The National Confidential Enquiry into Perioperative Deaths (NCEPOD) published its first report in 1990, examining all types of surgical operation. Among orthopaedic patients 'high-risk' groups had a 40–80% chance of deep vein thrombosis and a 1–10% chance of fatal PE. Among gynaecological patients the group at highest risk was those undergoing hysterectomy for malignant disease.

The NCEPOD identified risk factors for thromboembolism in gynaecological patients. These included age, obesity and previous deep vein thrombosis – the same as those the CEMD had identified for caesarean section. The Royal College of Obstetricians and Gynaecologists (RCOG) formed a small working party to decide what to do about this.

The RCOG takes action

The working party focussed on gynaecological surgery, caesarean section and pregnant women with a history of thromboembolism. Its report, published in 1995, was a model of clarity. It grouped women into low-, medium- and high-risk groups and recommended appropriate action for each group. Its recommendations for gynaecological surgery and caesarean section were kept separate, and each set was summarised on a single page – the classic 'one side of A4' (see Figures 9.3 and 9.4). Soon laminated photocopies of the appropriate page were seen in the anaesthetic rooms of operating theatres up and down the country.

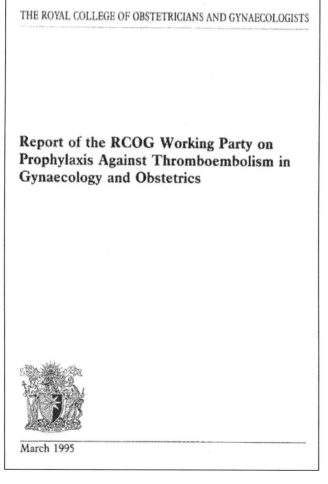

THE ROYAL COLLEGE OF OBSTETRICIANS AND GYNAECOLOGISTS

Report of the RCOG Working Party on Prophylaxis Against Thromboembolism in Gynaecology and Obstetrics

March 1995

Figure 9.3 The 1995 RCOG report

LOW RISK – Early mobilisation and hydration

☐ Elective caesarean section – uncomplicated pregnancy and no other risk factors

MODERATE RISK – Consider one of a variety of prophylactic measures

☐ Age > 35 years

☐ Obesity (> 80 kg)

☐ Para 4 or more

☐ Gross varicose veins

☐ Current infection

☐ Pre-eclampsia

☐ Immobility prior to surgery (> 4 days)

☐ Major current illness, e.g. heart or lung disease cancer; inflammatory bowel disease; nephrotic syndrome

☐ Emergency caesarean section in labour

HIGH RISK – Heparin prophylaxis +/– leg stockings

☐ A patient with 3 or more moderate risk factors from above

☐ Extended major pelvic or abdominal surgery, e.g. caesarean hysterectomy

☐ Patients with a personal or family history of deep vein thrombosis; pulmonary embolism or thrombophilia; paralysis of lower limbs

☐ Patients with antiphospholipid antibody (cardiolipin antibody or lupus anti-coagulant)

Figure 9.4 Risk assessment chart from the 1995 RCOG report

The importance of consensus

The RCOG report also summarised the CEMD's findings and previous recommendations, along with recent research including a guideline on pregnancy-associated thrombosis published in 1993 by the British Society of Haematology (BSH). This had reviewed the research in detail and allayed concerns about safety of heparin in pregnancy. Heparin is a powerful anticoagulant which has to be given by injection, and the RCOG felt able to recommend its use to prevent thromboembolism in women at highest risk.

The first reference in the BSH guideline was the CEMD Report for 1982–4, which had recommended 'serious consideration of prophylactic anti-coagulant therapy'. In turn, the CEMD Report for 1988–90 strongly endorsed the BSH guideline, and the CEMD reproduced in full the RCOG recommendations in its Report for 1991–3, published in 1996. Such a unanimous message could hardly fail to get across to working clinicians.

This interaction shows how the CEMD would work from then on. The CEMD's findings would stimulate research and its recommendations would be built on by other organisations. Today the first reference in many scientific papers is a CEMD Report, and the CEMD's recommendations have formed the basis for official guidelines.

The first success

The 1995 RCOG report came too late to affect the CEMD figures for 1994–6, which showed a rise in deaths from PE after caesarean section to a new high of 15. In the next report, however, however, they fell dramatically (see Figure 9.5). Only four women died, including one at very high risk who weighed 150 kg (23 stone).

Nevertheless, despite the gratifying reduction in deaths after caesarean section, PE was still the leading direct cause of maternal death by a considerable margin in 1997–9. It caused 13 deaths during pregnancy and 10 after vaginal delivery. The Report therefore recommended risk assessment at vaginal delivery similar to that at caesarean section. Women at moderate risk, it said, should receive subcutaneous heparin until they left hospital and those at the highest risk (women with a past history of thromboembolism) should receive heparin for six weeks after delivery.

Clinical freedom

The question was, would this advice be heeded? Risk assessment in the anaesthetic room or operating theatre was one thing. Risk assessment of every woman having a baby was quite another. Would doctors and midwives across the country follow the recommendations of a small group of special-ists? One of medicine's most cherished traditions was clinical freedom. Expert groups and Royal Colleges might issue guidance, but it was up to individual

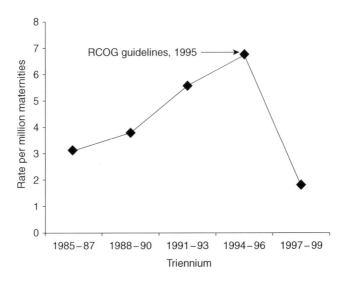

Figure 9.5 Death rate from thromboembolism after caesarean section, 1985–99

doctors to read it and decide for themselves whether to take the advice or ignore it.

Times, however, were changing. In 1983 the BMJ published an editorial entitled 'The End of Clinical Freedom'. The editorial was about the management of heart attacks, but it addressed a much wider issue and did not mince its words: 'Clinical freedom is dead, and no-one should regret its passing. Clinical freedom was the right – some seemed to believe the divine right – of doctors to do whatever in their opinion was best for their patients.' It ended with a flourish: 'Clinical freedom should have been strangled long ago, for at best it was a cloak for ignorance and at worst an excuse for quackery. Clinical freedom was a myth that prevented true advance.'

That polemic, written by J. R. Hampton, a professor of cardiology in Nottingham, was ahead of its time, but only by a few years. In 1989 a new type of standard textbook appeared. *Effective Care in Pregnancy and Childbirth* was written by 98 authors from 13 countries. The book featured a compilation of objective evidence from randomised trials and other high-quality research. The *British Journal of Obstetrics and Gynaecology* hailed it as 'probably the most important book in obstetrics to appear this century' in an editorial – which, interestingly, included extensive quotes from a book by Richard Asher.

By 1992 the phrase 'evidence-based medicine' had become part of the medical vocabulary and doctors were beginning to feel comfortable with the idea of following guidelines. The RCOG Working Party Report of 1995 avoided using that emotive word, though actually the RCOG had produced its first clinical guideline in 1994. Based initially on expert opinion, in 1996 the RCOG guidelines became 'national evidence-based guidelines' funded by the Department of Health. The tradition of clinical freedom had come to an end.

Its passing, however, was regretted by some, including Hampton himself. In 2010 the *International Journal of Epidemiology* reprinted his 1983 BMJ editorial along with admiring articles from other epidemiologists. It asked Professor Hampton, by then Emeritus, to contribute, and he did so in fine style. Having noted the inconsistency of 'evidence-based (which we ought to call opinion-based) proscriptive guidelines', he wrote, 'We need to change medical culture in such a way that doctors can use their opinions about published evidence to select the best treatment for each individual patient. We need a return to clinical freedom.'

Effective guidelines

Professor Hampton had a point, and in 2010 clinicians were already using their opinions. Some national guidelines led to action but others were – to put it kindly – unnecessarily complicated. In 2008 the National Institute for Health and Clinical Excellence (NICE) published a guideline called *Antenatal Care: Routine Care for the Healthy Pregnant Woman*. It totalled 457 pages – longer than the standard textbooks of the 1930s, which, far from being restricted to healthy women, covered the whole of obstetrics and gynaecology.

The RCOG guidelines, by contrast, were practical and more likely to be followed. The 1997–9 CEMD Report, published in 2001, had already shown that clear advice, succinctly communicated, could save the lives of women undergoing caesarean section. The next step was to extend its benefits to all pregnant women.

In January 2004 the RCOG produced a more comprehensive guideline entitled *Thromboprophylaxis during Pregnancy, Labour and after Vaginal Delivery*. This landmark publication was only 13 pages long. It began by quoting the 1997–9 CEMD Report, which had shown that all the women who died from PE after vaginal delivery had been either overweight or over the age of 35 years.

It also pointed out that pregnancy itself causes a tenfold increase in the risk of thromboembolism. During pregnancy levels of clotting factors in the blood increase because after birth, bleeding has to be controlled by a combination of uterine contraction and blood clotting. The clot consists of a protein, fibrin, formed from a soluble precursor, fibrinogen. By late pregnancy the circulating levels of fibrinogen have doubled, increasing the risk of thrombosis in susceptible women.

The risk is further increased by age and obesity – two factors which have changed in recent years (see Chapter 10). In 1993 the proportion of British women classed as obese was 16% but 10 years later it was 23%. The average age of a woman giving birth has also risen: the percentage aged over 35 rose from 8% in 1988–90 to 18% in 2002. Other risk factors identified by the RCOG guideline included varicose veins, previous thrombosis and medical conditions such as thrombophilia. Also listed were long-haul air travel, surgical operations, prolonged labour and dehydration due to excessive vomiting of pregnancy.

This long list meant that risk assessment was necessary not only at the beginning of pregnancy, but also later on. The guideline described preventive measures including drugs and compression stockings, and tests for suspected thrombosis, such as Doppler ultrasound and MRI scans.

Further success

The effects of the new RCOG guideline, published in 2004, were seen in the CEMD Report for 2006–8, but meanwhile deaths from thromboembolism rose again in the 2003–5 Report (see Figure 9.5). Two-thirds of those women received substandard care. Risk factors were not recognised or acted upon, and symptoms in at-risk women were inadequately investigated. Morbidly obese women (those with a BMI above 40) were given heparin in inadequate doses and the Report called for new guidelines for this group.

In 2006–8, however, the picture changed. As a result of the new RCOG guideline, the number of deaths from thromboembolism fell to 18, the lowest-ever total. Still, that number could – and should – have been lower. Substandard care was still occurring, particularly in minority ethnic groups and women with psychiatric problems or learning difficulties. The chapter concluded: 'A distressing feature is the over-representation of vulnerable women. The many pressures on the maternity services are no excuse for providing substandard service to women who require care in the true sense of the word.'

The bigger picture

Although the story of thromboembolism has been about one particular cause of maternal death, it also reveals a bigger picture of changing attitudes

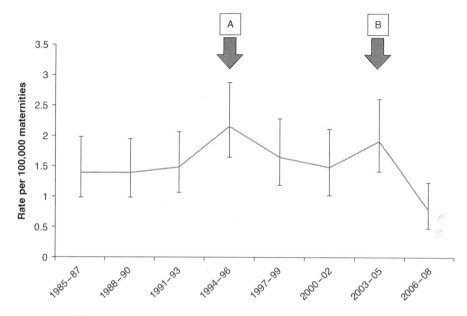

Figure 9.6 Overall death rate from thromboembolism, 1985–2008
Redrawn from "Saving Mothers' Lives: Reviewing maternal deaths to make motherhood safer 2006–2008"
A=The 1995 RCOG report (Figure 9.3)
B= The 2004 RCOG Guideline No 37, "Thromboprophylaxis during pregnancy, labour and after vaginal delivery".

and knowledge. The tradition of bed rest survived enlightened challenges for 200 years before fading away in the 1980s, partly because women began to question it. At first the CEMD merely recorded the resulting fall in mortality, but, as deaths became fewer, its role became more important.

The CEMD highlighted issues that would otherwise have gone unrecognised, motivated others to take action and demonstrated that targeted guidelines can save lives. The dramatic changes in the three-year intervals between well-publicised Reports may well have helped to produce the happy ending to this chapter. But motivation needs frequent reinforcement and in future the challenge will be to continue to engage the network of organisations – and the vast number of individuals – who contributed to that success.

10 PREGNANCY AND ILLNESS

Pregnant women can fall sick and women with chronic disease can become pregnant. Today in developed countries very few illnesses are fatal in women under 50, but sadly some are. A pregnant woman in the UK is now more likely to die of intercurrent disease than of the pregnancy itself. This is mainly because deaths from complications of childbirth have become rare, but there are other, more disturbing reasons. Risk factors for some diseases have increased and Confidential Enquiries into Maternal Deaths (CEMDs) have revealed substandard management of non-obstetric conditions, particularly among women living in difficult social circumstances.

Indirect deaths

The CEMD Reports have always included deaths which were not due directly to pregnancy, but it took many years for the impact of non-obstetric conditions to be fully recorded. From the beginning cardiac disease had its own chapter. The 1955–7 Report also mentioned that the 1957 Asian flu epidemic had caused 28 deaths – a higher-than-expected number – showing that pregnant women were at increased risk.

Other diseases, however, were not discussed until 1961–3, when a 'Miscellaneous' chapter appeared. The 1967–9 Report introduced a chapter on 'Deaths from Associated Causes' such as suicide, cancer, epilepsy and asthma. That chapter steadily expanded until 1976–8, when the terminology was revised by international agreement and associated deaths were subdivided into two groups, 'Indirect' and 'Fortuitous'.

'Indirect' deaths were defined globally as 'those resulting from a pre-existing disease or from a disease which developed during pregnancy and did not have a direct obstetric cause but was aggravated by the physiological effects of pregnancy'. (The CEMD decided also to include diseases whose management was changed by pregnancy.) 'Fortuitous' deaths were 'those unrelated to pregnancy or not aggravated by it'. From 1982–4 onwards each group had its own chapter in the Reports and in 1997–9 the name 'Fortuitous' was changed to 'Coincidental'.

The distinction between 'Indirect' and 'Coincidental' is not always straight-forward. All deaths from cardiac disease are classed as 'Indirect' because pregnancy puts a strain on the heart, but sometimes research is needed to find out if a disease is affected by pregnancy. Only a few cancers, for example, are influenced by placental hormones, and it takes time for the behaviour of a new disease such as COVID-19 to become clear.

'Coincidental' deaths may also need to be examined. When the 'Fortuitous' classification was introduced in 1976–8 it included road traffic accidents, but, after seat belts became compulsory in the 1980s, it became clear that some pregnant women were reluctant to use them. Advice on how to wear them safely became one of the important public health messages included in the CEMD Reports.

Improved reporting

In the early years of the CEMD, reporting of both 'Direct' and 'Indirect' deaths was incomplete. The 1952–4 Report included 1,094 deaths from 'Direct' causes and 361 from 'Associated' causes, while the Registrar General's figures were 1,403 and 409 deaths, respectively. By 1976–8, however, both systems were recording almost identical numbers of 'Direct' deaths, while 'Associated' deaths were difficult to compare because of the changes in terminology. The number of 'Indirect' deaths reported to the CEMD reached its lowest point in 1982–4 and then rose steadily (see Figure 10.1). Most of the increase was due to better reporting (in statistical parlance, 'improved ascertainment'), and, by the year 2000, the CEMD at last had an accurate picture of 'Indirect' maternal deaths across the UK.

As shown in Figure 10.1, 'Indirect' deaths outnumbered 'Direct' deaths from 1997–9 onwards. In 2006–8 there came a welcome reduction in both categories but 'Indirect' deaths still accounted for 60% of the total. They were due to a wide variety of diseases, many of which, such as asthma and HIV infection, caused no more than one or two deaths every year. A small number of conditions, however, made major contributions to maternal mortality. By far the most important of these was heart disease.

Heart disease

Pregnancy makes extra demands of the heart. The normal cardiac output is about five litres of blood per minute, but it rises by about 40% in pregnancy due to increases in both the heart rate and the amount pumped with each beat. Half of the increase occurs in the first 8 weeks (causing the bloom in the

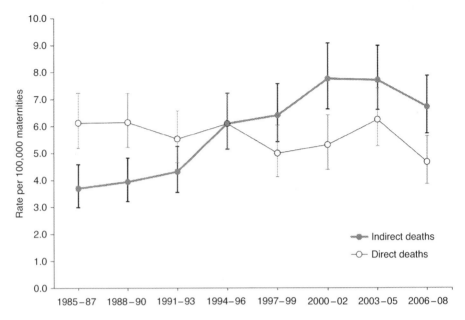

Figure 10.1 Rates of 'Indirect' and 'Direct' deaths, 1985–2008. Redrawn from data in the CEMD Reports.

skin which is hard to conceal from experienced eyes) and the maximum is reached by 30 weeks. During labour there is a further 50% rise as the uterine muscle squeezes blood back into the circulation, and this happens again just after the birth. It takes about 2 weeks for cardiac output to return to normal. A healthy heart can cope with these changes, but disease brings substantial risks.

Rheumatic heart disease

During the first 50 years of the CEMD the pattern of heart disease in Britain changed dramatically. In the 1950s the predominant type was rheumatic heart disease, now regarded as a disease of poverty. It has become rare in high-income countries but still affects an estimated 15.6 million people worldwide. The condition is an after-effect of rheumatic fever, a complication of streptococcal (and other) throat infections which affect mainly children between the ages of 5 and 15.

Acute rheumatic fever is an inflammatory response that develops one to five weeks after the infection. It causes pain in the joints (hence the name) and affects the heart less frequently but more seriously. As the nineteenth-century

French physician Ernst-Charles Lasègue memorably wrote, 'it licks at the joints, but bites at the heart'. Damage to the heart valves may take years to develop. The mitral valve, through which blood from the lungs enters the left ventricle, is most at risk. Tightening of the valve (mitral stenosis) leads to long-term stress on the heart and lungs, and an acute build-up of lung fluid can result in sudden death.

The 1950s

Mitral valve disease killed 96 women in 1952–4, and rheumatic disease of the other valves killed 12 more. Non-rheumatic heart disease caused another 13 deaths. The total of 121 deaths from heart disease was not far behind the leading causes of 'Direct' death in that Report. The cardiac chapter makes particularly sad reading. More than 50% of the women who died were in their twenties and most of them were having their first baby. Forty-four women died in labour or within 24 hours after birth.

An avoidable factor was present in at least 40 of the 121 deaths. Nineteen women with known heart disease had been booked for home delivery and 18 had refused to attend hospital at all, often because they had other children to look after and felt safe because they had given birth before. Mitral valve disease, however, is slowly progressive and the Report warned that 'a safe delivery in her earlier years is not necessarily any guarantee of a mother's safety in pregnancy in later years'.

In the next Report little seemed to change. Eleven of the women who died had given birth at home or in a small maternity home and 'in every case this unwise arrangement contributed directly and considerably to the fatal result'. Many women, however, died in hospital despite careful supervision. Nine died after caesarean section, leading the Report to conclude: 'The danger of Caesarean Section in pregnant women suffering from cardiac disease would appear to have been confirmed.' This statement is far from evidence-based by today's standards, as no valid comparison had been made with normal birth.

The streptococcus retreats

With the benefit of hindsight we can see that already in 1955–7 the picture was starting to improve. Deaths from heart disease had fallen by almost 20% since the previous Report, with a 40% drop among women aged 29 or under. These changes were entirely due to a reduction in rheumatic heart disease. Table 10.1 shows how the fall continued into the 1960s.

After 1966 the Reports no longer listed rheumatic heart disease systematic-ally. In 1970–2 it caused 16 deaths, mainly of older women with large families, and thereafter no more than 2–3 deaths per triennium. After 1988–90 it was

Table 10.1 Deaths from rheumatic heart disease and all cardiac disease, 1952–66

Triennium	Rheumatic heart disease	All cardiac disease
1952–4	108	121
1955–7	89	102
1958–60	54	66
1961–3	50	68
1964–6	22	43

not mentioned at all. Why did it disappear so completely? The usual answer is the introduction of penicillin – the first effective treatment for streptococcal throat infection. Young girls who received penicillin in the late 1940s would have been having their first babies in 1955–7, so the initial fall in mortality was indeed likely due to the new wonder drug.

Recently, however, experts have attributed the reduction in rheumatic fever to improved living conditions, with less overcrowding and better hygiene helping to limit the transmission of streptococci. We can see a parallel here with the reduction in puerperal sepsis at the same time (see Chapter 5), which was initially credited to antibiotics and then to improved obstetric and midwifery practice. In both cases, though, the reasons might be more complex. Epidemics continue to surprise us as the virulence of microorganisms waxes and wanes. We must be grateful that the streptococcus retreated in the 1950s, but we should bear in mind that we may not fully understand why.

Other Acquired Heart Disease

From 1961 the CEMD Reports divided heart disease into 'Congenital' and 'Acquired'. The latter group was initially dominated by rheumatic heart disease and, when this all but disappeared in 1972, there was sharp fall in the overall number of deaths from acquired heart disease. A close look at Table 10.2 shows the step change between 1970–2 and 1973–5.

The total continued to fall until the end of the 1980s. By then the main causes of acquired heart disease were coronary artery disease, myocardial infarction ('heart attack') and cardiomyopathy (a relatively rare disease of heart muscle), and it was these that accounted for the apparent increase in the 1990s shown in Figure 10.2. This will be discussed later, but first we shall look at congenital heart disease, which, as Figure 10.2 also shows, caused very few

Table 10.2 Deaths from acquired heart disease,
England and Wales, 1967–90

Triennium	Deaths from acquired heart disease
1967–9	34
1970–2	33
1973–5	14
1976–8	14
1979–81	12
1982–4	11
1985–7	9
1988–90	8

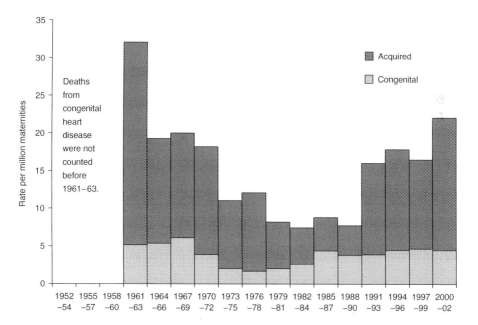

Figure 10.2 Rates of death from acquired and congenital heart disease, 1961–2002

maternal deaths in the 1970s before briefly becoming the main reported cause
of death from heart disease in the late 1980s.

Congenital Heart Disease

Congenital anomalies occur in around 2.4% of all births. Heart defects are a common anomaly found in up to 1% of babies, and they can be highly complex. Many include an incomplete septum between the atria or ventricles – a 'hole in the heart' – which allows mixing of oxygenated and deoxygenated blood, causing a so-called blue baby. Before treatment became available the child would grow up disabled by breathlessness. The heart became hypertrophied, leading to raised blood pressure in the lungs and problems with pulmonary blood flow. This combination was called Eisenmenger's syndrome after the Austrian physician who first described it in 1897. A woman living with this syndrome had a fifty-fifty chance of surviving pregnancy.

Early breakthroughs in treatment came from the USA. The first 'shunt' operation to compensate for the abnormal blood flow was performed in Johns Hopkins Hospital in 1944. That baby girl died months later but the operation became widely used and saved many lives. In 1956 the Nobel Prize for medicine was awarded to pioneers of cardiac catheterisation working in New York. The technique allowed research which transformed cardiology, and in the 1960s heart surgery began to expand rapidly across the world. Definitive treatment of heart defects became possible – though it was still a difficult and highly skilled procedure. Babies born with congenital heart disease (CHD) could survive and live a healthy life. A new question arose: how would they cope with pregnancy?

Risk-Taking and Counselling

The CEMD Report for 1961–3 was the first to differentiate CHD from other heart disease. It reported the deaths of 13 women at an average age of 23, of whom 7 had Eisenmenger's syndrome. In 1967–9 the total was again 13 but, during the 1970s, there were no more than 4 deaths from CHD in each Report. Women with the condition were strongly advised against pregnancy, advice the CEMD Reports reinforced.

In the 1980s, however, the number of deaths began to rise. By then corrective surgery had been available for more than 20 years and women who had survived this dangerous procedure in childhood believed they could cope with pregnancy. The CEMD remained cautious. The Report for 1985–7 recorded 10 deaths of women with CHD and commented, 'their cardiovascular system does not cope readily with the additional load of pregnancy and, especially, labour'. It recommended a team approach involving cardiologists, obstetricians and anaesthetists from the beginning of pregnancy, and birth in a unit which could deal with any cardiac surgical emergency.

For the next 15 years each Report included 9 or 10 deaths from CHD, often with avoidable factors. The 1988–90 Report commented that women with CHD 'seem particularly reluctant to accept medical advice concerning the dangers of childbearing'. Perceptively, it added that 'techniques for advising women with life threatening conditions could be improved'. Some doctors reacted badly when a woman said she still wanted to have a baby after being warned of the risks, and the 1994–6 Report commented that one woman 'may have been alienated from the highly specialised care she needed by advice not to get pregnant'. Women with CHD needed the best possible care if they were to survive pregnancy, and the Report advised, 'it must be made clear to the woman and her partner that whatever decision she makes will be respected'.

The advice seems to have been heeded. In 2003–5 and 2006–8 deaths from CHD were reduced to four in each triennium. Women who chose to become pregnant were receiving appropriate management from highly specialised teams, and lessons were being learned in a new way. Morbidity due to CHD was being reported to the UK Obstetric Surveillance Service (UKOSS), as discussed in Chapter 14.

Acquired Heart Disease in the 2000s
The year 1991 saw a sharp increase in acquired heart disease. This was probably due to improved ascertainment, but the numbers continued to rise. They almost doubled between 1991 and 2008, as shown in Table 10.3, and it seems very likely that this reflects not only better reporting, but also a genuine increase.

No single heart disease accounted for this. Autopsy diagnoses included myocardial infarction, ischaemic heart disease, cardiomyopathy and aortic dissection. In addition, from 2000–2 onwards some deaths were attributed to 'Sudden adult death syndrome' (SADS), diagnosed when death is presumed to be due to a cardiac arrhythmia after all other causes have been excluded. Sudden adult death syndrome caused 10 deaths in 2006–8. Six of the women who died were obese, with BMIs between 30 and 45, and in fact all the conditions classed as 'acquired cardiac disease', including SADS, share the same risk factors – obesity, smoking and age over 35 years. These factors often overlapped and many of the women also had a family history of heart disease and/or an underlying medical condition such as high blood pressure or diabetes.

Heart Disease and Social Class
The rising numbers of cardiac deaths therefore appear to reflect a change in women's general health. Britain's recent obesity epidemic has had a greater

Table 10.3 'Acquired' cardiac deaths, 1988–2008

Triennium	Deaths from acquired heart disease
1988–90	9
1991–3	27
1994–6	29
1997–9	35
2000–2	44
2003–5	48
2006–8	53

effect on women than on men. In 1980, 6% of men and 8% of women in the UK were obese. In 1998 the figures were 17% and 21%, and 20 years later they were 26% and 29%. Obesity today, like rheumatic fever in the 1940s, is associated with lower socio-economic class. The prevalence of childhood obesity is twice as high in the most deprived areas as in the least deprived areas.

Smoking is also related to social class. The overall rate of smoking has fallen to 12.5% of UK women, but rates are two and a half times higher in lower-paid than higher-paid occupations. Another risk factor, however, has a different relationship to socio-economic circumstances. The average age at childbearing has been rising in the UK, but more so in professional and managerial occupations. In 2019 almost 24% of births were to women aged over 35. These issues are discussed in more detail in Chapter 13.

Other diseases

Among the many other diseases causing 'Indirect' deaths, one group stands out – illnesses affecting the brain. Although the numbers are much lower than those for heart disease, when several CEMD Reports are aggregated together the totals make grim reading. In the 12 years from 1997 to 2008 a total of 84 women died from intracranial bleeding or blood clotting. Strictly speaking, though, cerebral haemorrhage, subarachnoid haemorrhage and cerebral thrombosis are diseases of the blood vessels rather than the brain itself, and the risk factors have been found to be the same as for diseases of the heart and blood vessels elsewhere in the body. Obesity is a risk factor for cerebral thrombosis and, less surprisingly, controlling high blood pressure will reduce the risk of cerebral haemorrhage.

Epilepsy

Epilepsy, however, is an entirely neurological disease. Between 1997 and 2008 it caused 47 maternal deaths, many of which could have been prevented. Pregnancy alters the blood levels of anti-epileptic drugs, but women living with epilepsy have become familiar with their condition and may not think of seeking further advice when they become pregnant. All too often their doctors and midwives are also unaware of the added risk. Treatment in pregnancy needs to be reviewed by a specialist who can advise on how to strike a balance between maintaining its effectiveness and minimising any risk to the baby.

Worryingly, the risk to the mother did not diminish across the years. In the 2006–8 Report epilepsy caused the deaths of 14 women. Three died from seizures, including one who died in the bath. The CEMD Reports have emphasised that women with epilepsy should be advised about the risks of bathing themselves and their babies while unattended. But the other 11 deaths did not involve fits. 'Sudden unexpected death in pregnancy' (SUDEP), which, like SADS, is presumed to be due to cardiac arrhythmia, occurs in chronic epileptics with poorly controlled seizures.

Of the 14 women in 2006–8, one-third had difficult social circumstances and were at particular risk, but only 6 of the 14 had received pre-pregnancy counselling. In one case the neurologist's advice was not followed and in another the neurology service took five months to respond to an urgent referral. Epilepsy in pregnancy should be perceived as a high-risk condition, and the challenge for the CEMD is getting this message across.

Cancer

Cancer is an age-related disease and is relatively rare in the reproductive years. It affects 1 in 1,000 women at the age of 30, and 2 in 1,000 at age 40. Malignant disease therefore causes few maternal deaths, and pregnancy does not worsen the progress of most cancers. The two which are affected are meningioma and melanoma. Meningioma, a tumour of the membranes covering the brain, has receptors for pregnancy hormones. Melanoma, a cancer of the skin, has a slightly worse prognosis in pregnancy than in non-pregnant women: it is unclear whether this is due to a direct effect of pregnancy or a delay in diagnosis. Each of these cancers caused seven late deaths in the 2006–8 Report. There were also two deaths from choriocarcinoma, the only cancer directly due to pregnancy.

Choriocarcinoma is a tumour of the placenta. It usually follows a miscarriage or 'molar pregnancy' (which consists of abnormal placental tissue), but it also affects 1 in 250,000 normal pregnancies. Today it is easily detected by an abnormally high pregnancy test and is curable by chemotherapy. In the early years of the CEMD it was fatal but in 1956 a medical milestone was passed when a woman in New York with advanced choriocarcinoma was treated with methotrexate – the first time any solid tumour had been cured in this way. Today there are three centres in the UK specialising in the treatment of gestational trophoblastic disease. They can generally cure the cancer, but their job is made much harder if prolonged bleeding after birth or miscarriage is not investigated properly.

The practical lessons on cancer in pregnancy were summed up by a special chapter in the Report for 2003–5. One of the messages was that 'pregnancy is not a contraindication for appropriate radiological investigations'. Modern X-rays pose no risk to the baby, and symptoms raising suspicion of cancer should be investigated in pregnancy as in the non-pregnant woman. This is discussed further in Chapter 14. The other message was that pregnant women should be encouraged to practise self-examination. In the past breast examination was a routine part of antenatal care, but this was abandoned in the 1980s as part of the trend to de-medicalise care in pregnancy.

Breast cancer and pregnancy

Breast cancer is the most common form of cancer in women in the UK, though not the leading cause of cancer deaths. (This is still lung cancer despite the fall in smoking among women.) Breast cancer is not directly affected by pregnancy, but the diagnosis of early cancer may be delayed by the normal changes of pregnancy and lactation. Five deaths were reported in 2006–8, three of which were classed as 'Coincidental' because the women already had advanced disease before pregnancy.

There is, however, an intriguing epidemiological link between pregnancy and breast cancer. Full-term pregnancy reduces a woman's risk of breast cancer later in life. The younger she is when she has her first baby, the lower her lifetime risk. Breast feeding adds little or no further protection and the effect disappears after the age of 35. The risk seems to be linked to the ovarian hormones produced during the menstrual cycle but, disappointingly, suppressing ovulation with the contraceptive pill does not reduce breast cancer risk. Some day, perhaps, a way will be found to mimic the effect of full-term pregnancy on the mammary gland, but that day seems far in the future.

Can indirect deaths be reduced?

The CEMD's increasing emphasis on 'Indirect' deaths has had far-reaching effects. It helped to give birth to a new specialty combining medicine and obstetrics – but only after a very long gestation. In 1962 Dr Cyril Barnes, formerly an assistant physician at Queen Charlotte's Hospital, London, published a textbook, *Medical Disorders in Obstetric Practice*. The book went through five editions and was translated into several languages. Barnes' successor as Britain's leading authority on the subject was Dr Michael de Swiet, whose name is now part of the book's title. He became a CEMD assessor in 1991 and remained as the sole physician assessor to the Enquiries while the number of reports of 'Indirect' deaths steadily rose and overtook 'Direct' deaths. In 2000 he was joined by Dr Catherine Nelson-Piercy. They worked together in the CEMD until 2005, and both of them pressed for the establishment of a new national specialty.

Today there are specialists in obstetric medicine in centres around the country. Their specialist society, the MacDonald Club, founded in 1975 and named after a far-sighted nineteenth-century obstetric physician, has evolved into the MacDonald Obstetric Medicine Society. There is an official subspecialty training programme, and training can be acquired through either the Royal College of Physicians or the Royal College of Obstetricians and Gynaecologists. For many years obstetrics and gynaecology has been perceived as a surgical specialty, and the correction of that bias can only benefit pregnant women with medical problems.

But such highly specialised care will reduce the number of 'Indirect' deaths only if there is first-class liaison between specialists, maternity teams and general practitioners (GPs). Detection of early disease is the special skill of GPs, but much of the responsibility for antenatal care has now been passed to midwives. Pregnant women are likely to discuss new symptoms or existing medical conditions with the maternity team, who must know when to refer. Their biggest challenge lies in providing high-quality care to women living in deprived circumstances – as highlighted by the number of avoidable deaths from epilepsy.

The role of the CEMD will continue to be to count 'Indirect' deaths and to identify patterns of substandard care which would otherwise pass unnoticed. Attention to these deaths was slow to develop, but the Enquiries eventually gave a complete picture, and this has been enhanced by the developments described in Chapter 14. A downward trend in 'Indirect' deaths may have begun but if it is to be maintained, continuing vigilance will be vital.

11 MATERNAL DEATH DUE TO ANAESTHESIA

Anaesthesia is a young specialty and obstetric anaesthesia is even younger, as this chapter will show. Before looking at deaths caused by anaesthesia in maternity practice in the UK, the history relevant to obstetrics will be summarised, including how anaesthetics were given and who administered them. The key events in the development of anaesthesia are listed in Table 11.1.

The development of anaesthesia

The initial agent used in 1846 was nitrous oxide, followed shortly afterwards by chloroform and ether (Figure 11.1). The introduction of anaesthesia was the breakthrough that allowed surgery to develop, and in turn anaesthesia itself improved as requirements increased and became more refined. The administration of anaesthetics in the UK was always in the hands of doctors. One of the early obstetric administrations was in 1853 when John Snow gave chloroform to Queen Victoria for the birth of her eighth child, Prince Leopold. She subsequently received it for the birth of Princess Beatrice. This royal approval was particularly important in making anaesthesia in midwifery morally acceptable, as doubts had been raised about the safety and propriety of rendering women unconscious (Figure 11.2).

Another key event relevant to obstetrics, first described in Germany in 1898, was the development of spinal anaesthesia – injection of local anaesthetic into the fluid around the spinal cord. It went on to have a chequered history because of cases of resultant paraplegia, eventually found to be caused by the method of re-sterilising needles in the 1950s. Spinal anaesthesia for caesarean section (CS) became commonplace only in the early 1990s.

Nitrous oxide (once called 'laughing gas') is an anaesthetic, but, in low concentrations, it is an analgesic – that is, it provides pain relief without loss of consciousness. Equipment to deliver a mixture of nitrous oxide and air was introduced in1933, enabling intermittent analgesia by inhalation during uterine contractions. The mixture, however, was hypoxic because it delivered only half the amount of oxygen normally required when breathing air (10.5%

Table 11.1 Events in the development of anaesthesia related to obstetrics

Year	Event
1846	First administration of general anaesthesia for surgery in the USA and, within weeks, in the UK.
1848	First death due to anaesthesia – a 15-year-old girl having chloroform for dental extraction in UK.
1893	The London Society of Anaesthetists founded. It became the Anaesthetic Section of the Royal Society of Medicine in 1908.
1898	First administration of successful clinical spinal anaesthesia, by August Bier of Germany.
1914–18	First World War. Advances in anaesthesia through treating troops.
1921	Extradural analgesia described by Fidel Pagés of Spain.
1922	First meeting of the Section of Anaesthetics of the British Medical Association.
1927	Spinal analgesia popularised by George Pitkin of the USA.
1930	Publication of the interim report of the Departmental Committee on Maternal Mortality and Morbidity.
1932	Association of Anaesthetists formed in the UK and Ireland.
1933	Robert Minnitt of Liverpool designs a machine to administer nitrous oxide and air for analgesia in labour.
1935	First examination of Diploma in Anaesthetics.
1937	First Professor of Anaesthetics in the UK – Sir Robert Macintosh, Oxford.
1947	Establishment of the Faculty of Anaesthetists of the Royal College of Surgeons of England (RCS).
1948	Introduction of the National Health Service (NHS). Anaesthesia is recognised as a specialty with full equality with other specialties.
1953	First examination for Fellowship of the Faculty of Anaesthetists (FFARCS).
1965	The Central Midwives Board approves a premixed 50% mixture of nitrous oxide in oxygen.
1969	The foundation of the Obstetric Anaesthetists' Association to promote the highest standards of care in every aspect of anaesthetic practice.
1988	The formation of the College of Anaesthetists, independent of the RCS
1992	Royal charter given. The Royal College of Anaesthetists formed.

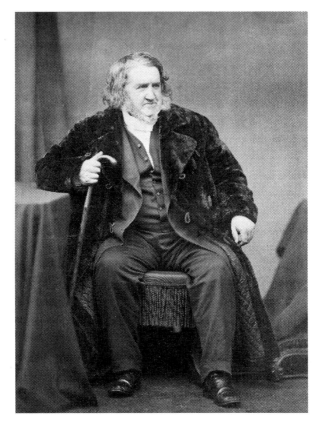

Figure 11.1 James Young Simpson (1811–70), professor of midwifery in Edinburgh, reported the first use of chloroform anaesthesia in 1847.

instead of 21%). This was rectified in the 1960s by developing cylinders of premixed nitrous oxide and oxygen (giving 50% oxygen) – although this is still called 'gas and air' by midwives and women! Self- administration by the mother is an important safety feature.

The many other important contributions from pharmaceutical and other companies have included numerous drugs, advances in anaesthetic machines, equipment for monitoring physiology, airway adjuncts and disposable single-use equipment. All have contributed to the modern safety of anaesthesia.

Of great significance too was the formation of societies enabling discussion and dissemination of information about drugs, equipment and methods of safe anaesthesia. These were the predecessors of the Royal College of

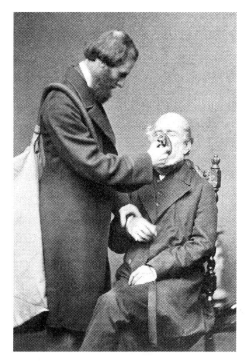

Figure 11.2 Joseph Clover (1825–82) administering anaesthesia from a reservoir bag held over his right shoulder. Clover weighed chloroform to produce an accurate mixture of 4.5% chloroform in air before going to the place of administration. Note that he is monitoring the patient's pulse.

Anaesthetists, which since 1992 has had responsibility for the maintenance and development of standards in the UK.

The safety of early anaesthesia

In the early years the isolated nature of anaesthetic practice and lack of broad data collection meant that information on anaesthesia's safety or otherwise was not widely available. The numbers of anaesthetic deaths in the Registrar General's annual reports were examined by William Stanley Sykes (an anaesthetist and crime writer) in his *Essays on the First Hundred Years of Anaesthesia*, published in 1960. In the first 100 years 24,378 deaths in England and Wales were due to or associated with anaesthesia, and in the first 50 years chloroform was invariably the agent associated with fatalities. The highest number (916) in a single year was in 1938, probably because of the increasing numbers of anaesthetics being given.

In 1946 there were 751 deaths and the total decreased by 200 annually until 1949. Sykes proposed three contributors to this improvement: first, widespread and easy availability of blood transfusion; second, the introduction of muscle relaxants combined with light anaesthesia; and third, more widespread availability of trained anaesthetists. Although this gives us useful background information, Sykes did not identify or comment on pregnant women.

The first collation of data pertinent to obstetric practice is in the chapter on 'anaesthetics and analgesics' in the Ministry of Health's *Interim Report on Maternal Mortality*, published in 1930. It covers the years 1911–29, when the overall maternal mortality rate from all causes was around 5 per 1,000 (1 in 226 maternities). Disquiet about the use of anaesthesia is evident from the fact that it warranted a separate chapter. A report from the Committee on the Training of Midwives had pointed out that 'it does not appear to be at all widely understood that the use of anaesthetics and other drugs is not without danger to mother and child in certain circumstances'.

The 1930 Report was a landmark document (see Chapter 2), but the chapter on anaesthetics gave no numbers or incidence nor any reasons for the mortality or morbidity. It called for a professional body to advise on these matters. Of great prescience, however, was the recommendation that the person giving the anaesthetic should not have divided duties. If the same person conducts the delivery, this distracts attention from the well-being of the mother and also increases the risk of sepsis. The danger of combined roles was not recognised in some other areas until 1983, when the operator-anaesthetist in dentistry was abolished.

The problems highlighted in the Report were addressed with more urgency after the inception of the NHS by national audit in the form of the Confidential Enquiry into Maternal Deaths (CEMD) (see Chapter 3). This will be discussed in more detail, but first more background information is needed.

Indications for anaesthesia

Many might wonder why anaesthesia is ever necessary for the natural process of childbirth. The overriding reason has been to ensure the safety of both mother and baby. An extreme example is placenta praevia, where the placenta completely covers the fully dilated cervix and the baby cannot be delivered vaginally without massive haemorrhage. Before anaesthesia and blood transfusion the mother and baby inevitably died. As monitoring of the health of both mother and baby has advanced, delivery by CS has been increasingly used.

Other reasons for pregnancy-related anaesthesia include forceps delivery, internal manipulations to correct a breech presentation, removal of a retained placenta in whole or in part, ectopic pregnancy and termination of pregnancy or of its retained products and procedures to deal with severe haemorrhage. Over time maternal comfort and the relief of pain in labour became more common indications for anaesthesia. In the early twentieth century this involved intermittent chloroform, or 'twilight sleep' with intramuscular drugs such as omnopon (an opiate later superseded by pethidine) and scopolamine. From the late 1960s onwards more use was made of epidural analgesia using local anaesthetics targeted at the pain pathways from the uterus and lower genital tract.

Anaesthetising the pregnant woman

It is important to note that there are major differences between anaesthetising a woman in advanced pregnancy compared to one who is not pregnant. At the end of pregnancy there is a physiological 40% increase in 'minute volume' (the amount of air breathed in and out of the lungs in each minute) and a comparable increase in cardiac output. These two factors cause a drastic reduction in the time that a woman can hold her breath (or not be ventilated) before she becomes hypoxic (short of oxygen). If she breathes 100% oxygen for a few minutes before anaesthesia, more time is available for the anaesthetist to gain control of her breathing, which has to be done rapidly if muscle relaxants are given. (These induce paralysis of all muscles, including the abdominal muscles, enabling surgical access to the uterus.) Normally the anaesthetist inserts a tube into the trachea, using a laryngoscope to visualise the vocal cords, and then applies artificial ventilation. The breast enlargement of pregnancy can make this more difficult.

Another special factor in late pregnancy is that, if the woman is laid flat on her back, the enlarged uterus will compress the major blood vessels (the aorta and inferior vena cava), compromising the blood flow to the uterus. To avoid this, she is partially tilted onto her left side, which also makes tracheal intubation more difficult by deviating the laryngeal aperture from the midline.

A further important physiological change involves the stomach. Relaxation of the lower oesophageal sphincter – the ring of muscle which keeps the stomach contents in place – and reduced motility of the stomach itself combine to cause gastric reflux. If this happens when the woman is paralysed, causing loss of the protective cough reflex, the stomach contents can enter the lungs with potentially fatal results.

All these problems are compounded in obesity, which has become increasingly common in the UK. These risk factors are well known to obstetric anaesthetists but were not always appreciated in earlier years. Additionally, pregnancy is the only situation where the anaesthetist is responsible for two patients – or more in a multiple pregnancy – simultaneously and on many occasions the stress is compounded by the need for a speedy response to an emergency. Cool heads and competent hands are required.

The early Confidential Enquiries

The preface of the first CEMD Report (1952–4) drew attention to the fact that anaesthesia was a primary or associated cause in nearly 1 in 20 of all maternal deaths. The aim was to raise awareness that maternal death occurs and to find ways of reducing mortality. Inhalation of stomach contents into the lungs was the major factor, causing 32 of the 49 deaths from anaesthesia.

Table 11.2 shows that, in each of the triennial reports from 1952 to 1984, women died from inhalation of gastric contents. This causes death either immediately by asphyxiation or later due respiratory failure from the effect of gastric acid on the lungs. The acid causes pneumonitis, leading to adult respiratory distress syndrome (ARDS) – a condition named Mendelson's syndrome after the American obstetrician who first described it in 1946. Tracheal intubation isolates the trachea from the oesophagus and prevents gastric contents from entering the lungs, but, at that time, most anaesthetists used a simple face mask to maintain an airway and administer inhalational anaesthetics.

The second triennial Report (1955–7) commented that 'it is a wise precaution to intubate the trachea when the stomach is thought to be full and where forceps delivery is to be undertaken in the lithotomy position'. The lithotomy position involves the woman lying on her back with full flexion of the legs, and this is more likely to precipitate regurgitation. The 1958–60 Report reinforced this point. The early Reports did not ascribe deaths to any particular anaesthetic agent. Those most used were ether, trichloroethylene, chloroform and cyclopropane, and there was one death after spinal anaesthesia. By the 1970s none of those inhalational agents was in regular use.

Table 11.2 Total maternal deaths and the numbers caused by anaesthesia in the years 1952 to 1966 in England and Wales. N/A = not identified in report

Years	Maternal deaths (n)	Anaesthetic deaths (n)	Anaesthetic deaths as % of maternal deaths	Death caused by inhalation of stomach contents (n)	Difficulty intubating trachea (n)
1952–4	1,094	49	4.8	32	N/A
1955–7	861	31	3.6	18	N/A
1958–60	742	30	4.0	17	3
1961–3	692	28	4.0	16	N/A
1964–6	579	50	8.6	26	0
1967–9	455	50	11.0	26	10
1970–2	343	37	10.4	16	3
1973–5	227	37	16.3	13	7
1976–8	217	40	18.4	14	16
1979–81	178	29	16.3	8	8
1982–4	138	18	13.0	7	10

The need for change

Table 11.2 also shows that the proportion of maternal deaths from anaesthesia steadily increased until at least the late 1970s. Although one might infer that anaesthesia was becoming more dangerous, or, at the very least, there was no improvement, we cannot tell without knowing how many anaesthetics were given. This information is not available but, because CS always requires anaesthesia, the rate of CS is an indicator of the number of anaesthetics. In 1964–6 the CS rate was 3.4% of all maternities. By 1982–4 it was 10.1% and by the end of the century it was 21%. However, it is not an exact reflection of the number of anaesthetics because there were more births in the early years and anaesthesia was often required for forceps delivery.

The Reports indicate that practice in the early years was quite different from that in the 1970s and after. In 1955–7, for example, 'in five, and possibly six, cases the anaesthetic was administered by a single-handed obstetrician' and in 1961–3 'anaesthesia (spinal anaesthesia for CS) appeared satisfactory but respiratory difficulties occurred before the operation was completed. By this time the anaesthetist was busy elsewhere and not immediately available'. These illustrations speak for themselves. It later became unthinkable that an anaesthetist would not be present throughout the procedure. Yet the very first Report had emphasised the need for an anaesthetist experienced in obstetric work to be available at night, when these emergencies often occur, as well as in the day.

In 1961–3 various measures were advocated to avoid gastric content inhalation. 'Failure to intubate the trachea was the commonest fault', said the Report, 'though this procedure alone is not an absolute safeguard'. One method was Sellick's manoeuvre, which involves firmly pressing the cricoid cartilage (just below the larynx) to flatten the oesophagus against the vertebral body behind. There is also mention of avoiding general anaesthesia by using local anaesthetic to block the pudendal nerves and numb the vagina for forceps delivery. This was commended but 'not too much should be expected of it' as two women who died had required general anaesthesia in a hurry because the pain relief was inadequate. Again in 1964–6 there were two deaths after pudendal block, but there were many more from inhaled stomach contents. In 1967–9 there was the first mention of giving, before anaesthesia, an oral antacid in the form of magnesium trisilicate, although one woman died despite it having been administered.

The formation of the Obstetric Anaesthetists Association in 1969 was a very useful forum where the deaths were discussed and views were exchanged on how to tackle problems. Magnesium trisilicate was unpopular with women because it was unpalatable and the CEMD Reports for 1970–2 and 1973–5 acknowledged that it was part of the solution but not a panacea. In all the deaths from aspiration of stomach contents, cricoid pressure was found to have been either not applied, ineffectually applied or released too early. It must be applied by an assistant familiar with the technique, who will not relax the pressure until the trachea is intubated.

The 1970s: identifying the problems

The 1973–5 Report therefore recommended that 'it is important that all con-cerned, anaesthetists, nursing staff and administrators, recognise that anaes-thetists require skilled help to deal with the hazard of inhalation of stomach contents'. At the hospital where I worked as a junior then, each time a different porter brought the woman to the operating theatre he had to be instructed how to perform the cricoid pressure and he was anxious to return to his other duties. By the late 1980s dedicated trained help was available.

The 1976–8 Report commented that the causes of anaesthetic maternal death were multifactorial. They were usually a combination of inexperience, low general standards of care in labour and in the operating theatre, and poor administrative practices in the form of unskilled assistance or isolation from fully equipped hospitals. That Report made the important instruction that 'an adequate drill for difficult intubation must be taught and put into practice by all who give anaesthetics for obstetric patients'.

The same Report added that 'the apparent obsession that an endo-tracheal tube must be passed even if to do so requires successive attempts by anaesthetists in ascending order of seniority is not rational'. Light anaesthesia was used for CS to avoid anaesthetising the baby, but the Report commented that deeper anaesthesia would prevent vomiting even without an endotracheal tube – and, poignantly, 'is less harmful to the neonate than having no mother'. The Report also noted that airway prob-lems were not the only cause of death. Four deaths were caused by misuse of drugs and two by accidents with apparatus, and there were four deaths from epidural analgesia.

By 1979–81 there continued to be deaths from airway difficulties and aspiration of gastric contents, but seven women died because of failure to provide appropriate post-operative care. Highlighting these deaths was cru-cial to the future of proper post-operative care provision in maternity units, where care should be comparable to that of patients recovering from surgery in other units or hospitals. There was one death from epidural anaesthesia. The essential role of anaesthetists in the management of severe bleeding was also acknowledged. Two deaths from this cause had highlighted the need for both obstetricians and anaesthetists to have a drill for the management of severe haemorrhage.

Looking back at Table 11.2, it is evident that, as deaths from aspiration of stomach contents reduced, deaths from difficulties in intubating the trachea increased. This is also seen in Table 11.3, which covers the maternal deaths from anaesthesia in the whole of the UK. The 1982–4 Report was the last that pertained to England and Wales. Its messages were depressingly similar to those in previous Reports, with continued deaths from airway problems and gastric acid aspiration. It commented that the recommended regimen of magnesium trisilicate had mostly been followed, which raised the question of whether the administration of a particulate antacid is safe. New drugs had been developed to reduce gastric acid production, and the Report suggested that H2 receptor antagonists such as cimetidine or ranitidene, as well as the buffering agent sodium citrate, might be a preferable way to raise the pH of stomach secretions. Equally essential are efforts to reduce the volume of stomach contents during labour.

It is depressing to summarise the first 30 years of Confidential Enquiries as demonstrating an increase in the proportion of maternal deaths due to anaesthesia. Deaths resulting from aspects of obstetric management had decreased, but there was no meaningful improvement in deaths from anaesthesia despite the repeated identification of gastric aspiration and difficulties with tracheal intubation as the most prominent causes.

1984–2002: The UK Reports

The first of the UK-wide Reports, however, showed early signs of improvement, as seen in Table 11.3.

Although more anaesthetics were being given, the proportion of deaths caused by anaesthesia was markedly lower than previously. 'Late' deaths – more than six weeks after the birth – are counted separately in the Reports, and the late deaths shown in column 2 in Table 11.3 were due to hypoxia causing serious brain damage that ultimately was not consistent with life. Intubation failures continued, even though difficult intubation drills were being practised and boxes were made up containing equipment that might be useful in case of difficult intubation.

Table 11.3 Total maternal deaths and the numbers caused by anaesthesia in the years 1985–2000 in the United Kingdom

Years	Maternal deaths (n)	Anaesthetic deaths (n)	Inhalation of stomach contents	Intubation problems	Spinal/Epidural management
1985–7	223	6 + 2 late	1	6	0
1988–90	238	4+1 late	1 + 1 late	1	1
1991–3	228	8	2	5	0
1994–7	268	1	0	0	1
1998–2000	242	3	1	1	1

Regional anaesthesia

The 1980s heralded a shift in methods of anaesthesia for CS. Many, if not most, units were frequently using epidural anaesthesia for pain relief in labour. This involves leaving a catheter in the epidural space to facilitate top-ups as the local anaesthetic wears off, and it was only a short step to increase the blockade from analgesia to more extensive anaesthesia that would enable CS. Such regional anaesthesia means that the woman remains awake and retains her protective laryngeal reflexes to prevent any regurgitated stomach contents from being aspirated to the lungs. The use of epidural anaesthesia also became commonplace for elective operations in obstetrics, giving the mother the bonus of seeing her baby at the moment of birth.

As mentioned earlier, the use of spinal anaesthesia only became common from the early 1990s. Spinal anaesthesia is a one-off injection directly into the cerebrospinal fluid that surrounds the spinal cord. A smaller volume and lower dose of local anaesthetic is required than for epidural and the onset of analgesia is more rapid, making spinal anaesthesia useful for emergencies as well as elective surgery. Both techniques require meticulous asepsis and reasonable technical expertise.

Complications that can result from either regional technique are infection, failure to locate the space to insert the local anaesthetic resulting in need for general anaesthesia, total spinal block resulting in profound hypotension (low blood pressure) and respiratory arrest. There can be drastic hypotension but with breathing maintained, and there can be headache, which sounds innocuous but can be miserable though it is curable.

As remaining awake for surgery has become more accepted, many women choose regional anaesthesia. This helps to reduce acid aspiration, as have the administration of sodium citrate and H2 receptor antagonists (taken orally) and reduced food intake in labour. There are logistical difficulties in administering such acid prophylaxis, but sodium citrate and H2 blockers are widely used before CS.

New advances and new problems

A crucial advance in the 1980s was that greatly improved monitoring became available (Figure 11.3). The pulse oximeter measures the oxygen saturation of haemoglobin in the blood and gives warning of hypoxia before the eye of the anaesthetist might detect cyanosis. Another great advance was capnography, which detects carbon dioxide in each inspired and expired breath. There should be no carbon dioxide in inspiration and around 5% in expired breath.

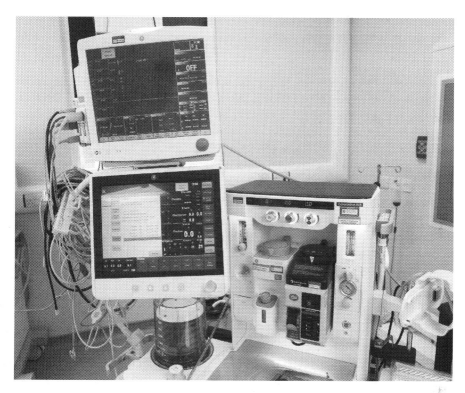

Figure 11.3 A modern anaesthetic machine in use in UK hospitals. Such machines have piped supplies of gases from a central source with back-up supplies from cylinders attached to the machine. The machine also has accurate flometers to deliver gases, vaporisers to incorporate accurate amounts of volatile anaesthetic agents, suction apparatus and a ventilator for artificial ventilation. Monitoring equipment includes that for cardiovascular variables (heart rate, ECG, blood and central venous pressures), respiratory variables (rate of breathing or artificial ventilation, inspired and expired ventilatory pressures and gas supplies) and indirect measurement of blood variables (oxygen saturation) and inspired and expired carbon dioxide values.
Photograph kindly provided by Professor T. H. Clutton-Brock

If, for instance, an endotracheal tube is misplaced in the oesophagus rather than the trachea, no cyclical change in carbon dioxide will be visible, and if cardiac output is reduced less carbon dioxide will reach the lungs. This monitoring was slower to be introduced in obstetrics than in general operating theatres, but it became accepted that there is no reason pregnant women should receive inferior monitoring.

If anaesthetic deaths are largely avoided by using spinal or epidural anaesthesia, is there any place for using general anaesthesia? There are few but definite contraindications to the regional techniques. These include coagulopathy (problems with blood clotting), which increases the risk that puncturing an epidural vein might cause a large haematoma (collection of blood), damaging nerves by pressure effects. Other contraindications are infection over the site of injection, which could be spread to the nervous system, severe haemorrhage, because low blood pressure can be worsened by blocking the sympathetic nervous system, or a neurological condition affecting the area to be blocked. Occasionally there is a failure to achieve a block at all, or only one that is inadequate to allow surgery. Naturally regional anaesthesia is also contraindicated if the woman is unwilling despite proper information and discussion.

Deaths from regional anaesthesia do occur, but rarely. They are largely due to inexperience and lack of training of the operator, as was apparent in the four cases in the 1976–8 triennium. Since then, there has been at most one case in each triennium.

One of the consequences of reduced use of general anaesthesia in obstetrics is that many anaesthetists are no longer experienced with it. This means that, when it is necessary, they are unfamiliar with the routine. Furthermore, the introduction of the laryngeal mask into anaesthesia means that anaesthetists in general are less experienced in the technique of intubation. The laryngeal mask is sited in back of the throat just over the larynx and is easily inserted, but it is not suitable for obstetric anaesthesia because it does not protect the airway from aspiration of regurgitated gastric contents.

Towards present day standards

Eventually – one has to say *eventually* because it took so long to see improvements – the tragedy of deaths from anaesthesia for obstetrics has been hugely reduced. The battle has been hard won by strategies of improved education and training, enhanced staffing of maternity units including trained assistants for anaesthetists and improved equipment and monitoring.

Table 11.4 illustrates the improvement in safety of anaesthesia for CS. For a woman in the year 2000 the risk of dying because of anaesthesia is 38-fold less than that in the mid-1960s. In other words, anaesthesia for CS is 6 times safer than in 1983 and 38 times safer than in 1964.

In the CEMD Report for the late 1990s there were few maternal deaths from anaesthesia, and the anaesthetic chapters took the opportunity to highlight areas of concern even when they were not the primary cause of death, in order to improve clinical practice.

Have the lessons highlighted by the Confidential Enquiries been taken on board, or has the impetus to maintain standards waned? The CEMD has

Table 11.4 Maternal risk of dying from anaesthesia for CS in three triennia from 1964 to 2002

Triennia	Maternities N	CS rate	CS n	Total anaesthetic deaths n	Deaths after anaesthetic for CS	Risk of death from anaesthesia for CS
1964–6	2,600,000	3.4%	88,400	50	32	1 in 2,763
1982–4	1,884,000	10.1%	190,284	19	11	1 in 17,299
2000–2	1,997,000	21.0%	419,370	7	4	1 in 104,842

always relied on its recommendations being taken up by other organisations, and *Guidelines for Obstetric Anaesthesia* was published by the Obstetric Anaesthetists Association (OAA) and the Association of Anaesthetists of Great Britain and Ireland (AAGBI) and *Standards of Good Practice* by the Royal College of Anaesthetists (RCA). At the end of the 1990s concerns about the rising CS rate led the Department of Health to commission an investigation by the Royal Colleges of Obstetricians, Midwives and Anaesthetists and the National Childbirth Trust. Its findings were published in 2001 as the *National Sentinel Caesarean Section Audit Report*, which covered the UK and concluded that compliance with standards in the OAA/AAGBI/RCA guidelines was high.

The Report looked at auditable standards. One was that acid prophylaxis should be administered prior to regional or general anaesthesia, and this was done in 90% of cases. Another was that the majority of CS should be performed with a regional block, and overall 77% of emergency and 91% of elective CS were performed using regional anaesthesia. Cross-matched blood facilities on site at all times were reported in 95% of maternity units. After CS 10% women required care in addition to routine post-operative care, and 91% of this care was provided in a high-dependency area within the maternity unit. These results confirmed the adherence to recommended standards and safe environs of maternity units.

To sum up, the fact that the Confidential Enquiry reports are read widely and have shown such a marked dramatic reduction in anaesthesia-related maternal deaths is worth celebrating. It took many years of persistent effort to achieve the safety standards we now take for granted. They are a good example of successful self-regulation by doctors and midwives.

12 PSYCHIATRIC ILLNESS

The risk of maternal death has cast a long shadow over the care of women during pregnancy and the postnatal period, but with the development of modern obstetric practice, mortality rates have plummeted in much of the Western world. However, in the context of this overall reduction, deaths associated with mental ill health have emerged as a prominent cause of maternal mortality. Between six weeks and one year after delivery, mental illness is now the leading cause of maternal death in the UK and Ireland.

How the Enquiries have addressed psychiatric deaths

The Confidential Enquiries into Maternal Deaths (CEMDs) have always included deaths due to mental disorder, but it was only in the 1994–6 Report that a specific chapter, led by a central psychiatric assessor, gathered these deaths together and discussed them in detail.

By the time of the 1997–9 Report the central psychiatric assessor was joined by an obstetrician with a special interest in substance misuse, bringing additional insights into deaths related to complex disadvantage – and frequently, comorbid physical ill health. In the two following reports, substance misuse psychiatry was represented among the team of authors. For the 2006–8 triennium, regional psychiatric assessors were appointed, and a second perinatal psychiatrist joined the central panel of assessors. Since then there has been robust representation from the ever-expanding family of perinatal psychiatrists from across the UK and Ireland.

Two groups of mental health-related deaths – maternal suicide and substance misuse – formed the backbone of all the Reports. The 1994–6 Report explored these and highlighted limitations which have, to some degree, continued to dog the Reports. First among these is the perennial problem of enumerating psychiatric deaths – the challenge of under-reporting. Deaths may not have been considered as having a psychiatric cause, and the reporting of late deaths relied on professionals with less connection to the Enquiries, so the deaths of many women are likely to have remained unknown. This continued to be a major problem until the introduction of record linkage to ensure greater comprehensiveness.

The second limitation, which remains to this day, is the paucity of psychiatric records submitted to the Enquiries. Assessors often have to divine the nature and quality of any psychiatric care from maternity or primary care records, hoping that these will include copies of assessment letters completed by mental health professionals. Not having the original notes to hand means the assessors risk doing a disservice to the treating teams by failing to reflect the quality of professional interactions. In contrast, one of the great strengths of the Enquiries has been its routine assessment of late deaths – the grouping into which most psychiatric mortality falls.

These limitations should not take away from the profound effect the Reports' specialist psychiatric chapters have had on the care of individual women and the provision of dedicated services across the UK. In the 1992–4 and subsequent Reports, led initially by Professor Channi Kumar and then by Dr Margaret Oates (two of the founders of modern perinatal mental health practice worldwide), the Enquiries have shone a light on the stories of women whose lives were lost to mental health-related causes. They have identified risk factors to aid clinical decision-making, informed and directed the expansion of specialist perinatal mental health service provision in the UK and beyond, and established psychiatric illness on a par with physical ill health in the minds of maternity professionals and service commissioners. In short, the Enquiries have had a profound effect on the care of women with mental disorder and their infants.

Indirect versus direct deaths

A major change to the international classification of maternal death by suicide took place in 2012 when the World Health Organization recategorised suicide, whatever the underlying psychiatric diagnosis, as a 'Direct' cause of maternal death. While the reclassification may be controversial and has led to a questioning of the usefulness of maintaining the distinction, it does reflect the importance the UK and Ireland Enquiries have long placed on psychiatric causes and, it is hoped, has acted as a spur to raise awareness and reduce under-reporting in the UK and other areas of the world.

What the Enquiries tell us

The women who died
Recommendations for improving care begin with the Enquiries' careful examination of socio-demographic characteristics, timing and mode of death,

mental health diagnosis and level of care received. Most of the women have had more than one baby. We have known from the earliest Enquiries that women who die by suicide are less likely to be socially deprived than those who die through substance misuse. This echoes research and historical observation demonstrating that women from all strata of society have a similar risk of experiencing the most severe forms of post-partum mental illness.

Ascribing diagnosis for the women who died by suicide has proved more difficult, given the frequent lack of psychiatric records available to the Enquiries. Nevertheless in most cases there has been enough information for assessors to reach confident conclusions. From the outset the most common diagnosis was of depressive disorder, either recurrent or newly arising in the perinatal period. Psychosis (most commonly depressive psychosis) has been diagnosed in 20–40% of women dying by suicide. A small but consistent proportion of women in this group have a primary diagnosis of substance misuse. Although particularly important in terms of prevention, the numbers of women with bipolar disorder or previous post-partum psychosis are low.

Overall suicide rates are reduced in pregnancy and the post-partum period when compared to other times. However, the post-partum reduction is much less marked and, where women have an underlying mental illness, their risk is significantly elevated. This is borne out in the timing of suicide reported in the Enquiries, and matches the known increased risk of admission to psychiatric hospital in the weeks and month after birth, which remains elevated for at least two years post-partum.

First reported in the 1997–9 Report, several subsequent Enquiries have defined the highest level of psychiatric care received by women during the episode of illness leading to their suicide. Surprisingly, the proportion of women receiving psychiatric care has fallen – from 85% in 1997–9 to 60% in 2017–19. This is most likely explained by reduced reporting in earlier years and the absence of data linkage. However, there has been a slow but steady increase in numbers of women who have been engaged with specialist peri-natal mental health teams. Given the very rapid expansion of services in the UK over the past five years, it is perhaps surprising that the change is not more marked.

The women who lost their lives through substance misuse died most commonly by accidental overdose or other medical complications related to their use. In the main, they had experienced greater social deprivation and complex adversity.

In its recommendations the 1994–6 Report highlighted twin themes which have dominated all subsequent reports – the need for changes to individual clinical practice and the requirement for structural change in the provision of dedicated mental health services for childbearing women. In addition, the Enquiries recognised substance misuse as a significant contributor to death, not only by suicide and accidental overdose, but also through its impact on general health and maternity care.

Lessons for clinical practice

Prevention of illness occurrence or reccurence

There is a clear opportunity for preventive interventions in perinatal mental health. Based on the first case descriptions, the Enquiries recommended universal screening for a history of mental disorder. The 1997–9 Report advised that this should take place at booking. This has now become standard practice in maternity services. Screening questions to identify significant past mental illness and evidence of current depression and anxiety are usually incorporated into the booking documentation.

In parallel, the 2000–2 Enquiry highlighted the importance of good communication between primary care and maternity services regarding relevant mental health history. Subsequent reports emphasised a similar duty of information-sharing by maternity and mental health services.

Recognising how often opportunities to intervene were missed, a repeated message has been that women identified as having a history of significant mental disorder should have psychiatric assessment during pregnancy. They should be counselled about their risk of recurrence in this and future peripartum periods, and a management plan for their care should be shared with them and with all professionals involved in their care. The use of late pregnancy mental health management plans has now become universal in specialist perinatal mental health services.

In 2017 the Enquiries published a morbidity audit in which women who had a prior diagnosis of bipolar disorder or post-partum psychosis were followed through a subsequent pregnancy and post-partum period. This broadened the opportunity to examine preventive interventions (or their lack) in more detail. The report outlined a number of 'amber flags' – cautions around risk of recurrence – including the importance of a history of any psychotic disorder as indicator of early post-partum risk and the need to consider personal and family history and pattern of occurrence and reoccurrence in risk evaluation. It also emphasised a triad of preventative measures to reduce future risk (Figure 12.1).

Acute risk assessment and management

There have been repeated messages in the Enquiries about the need to take into account the distinctive patterns of illness progression in the perinatal period

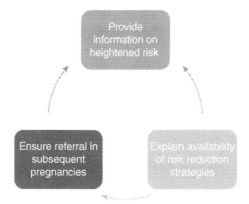

Figure 12.1 Preventive triad for women at heightened risk in future pregnancies or postpartum periods

when carrying out acute assessments or implementing risk-management strategies. Several reports identified a failure to make comprehensive assessments, to complete mental state evaluation, to recognise escalating symptoms or to act on any suicide risk identified.

The 2006–8 Report emphasised the need to modify risk assessment to account for the distinctive nature of perinatal mental illness. The next Report 'red flagged' the presence of significant change or emergence of new symptoms as indicators of suicide risk. It also specified two other 'red-flag' indicators of suicide risk: new expressions or acts of violent self-harm, and new or persistent expressions of incompetence as a mother or estrangement from the infant. It suggested that review by a senior clinician was essential for women with concerning symptom presentations, and it provided guidance on what presentations should trigger consideration of in-patient care in a mother and baby unit (MBU).

The 2014–16 Report broadened concern regarding all self-harm acts, which should be regarded as unusual in pregnancy or the early post-partum period, and should prompt referral, ideally to a perinatal mental health service.

The important contribution of partners and families to the support of women with mental illness has been recognised as a core factor in several Reports. Three broad messages have emerged: (i) the need to listen to relatives' concerns, remembering that they will know the woman better than any professional; (ii) the importance of educating relatives about the significance and serious nature of perinatal mental illness so they know when to be concerned;

and (iii) a caution that relatives are not mental health professionals and should not be asked to manage risk at an inappropriate level.

Reports have cautioned that women with multiple adversities may be particularly vulnerable and that disengagement from care or alterations in presentation are potential indicators of a worsening mental state. Their risk assessment is complex and there is a particular need for careful risk evaluation in women with substance misuse, with pregnancy or infant loss or with a history of complex trauma.

Prescribing issues

The decision to continue or stop prescribed medication during pregnancy or breastfeeding is an important aspect of risk management. The 2014–16 Report focussed on the tendency to prioritise potential risks over benefits, and failure to give women and families a balanced account to enable them to make informed decisions about their care (see also Chapter 14).

A new message on prevention in relation to prescribing emerged in the most recent report (2017–19). Women who had stopped medication during pregnancy were not re-evaluated after the birth – at a time of increased risk – for recommencement. The new recommendation suggests that any woman who had discontinued medication before or during pregnancy should be assessed early in the post-partum period regarding the need to restart.

Early reports discussed the type of medication and advised strongly against treating postnatal depression with progesterone – a practice that was commonplace but lacked any empirical evidence. This led to a clear change in prescribing practices from the early 2000s.

Lessons for service organisation

No matter what improvements are made to individual practice, poorly designed systems surrounding the practitioner and the pregnant woman will continue to limit the provision of effective care. It is interesting that, of the three mental health recommendations in the 1994–6 Report, one related to clinical practice, one to service provision and one to improving the Enquiries' analysis of case reports.

Its recommendation for service provision was that in each area a clinician should be identified who would be responsible for providing a perinatal mental health service. In the mid-1990s such services were present in only a handful of larger cities in England and barely at all in the other nations of the UK. In subsequent reports, there was an evolving pattern of guidance for service development, beginning in 1997–9 with recommendations that an

MBU and specialist community team should be available to every woman who required them. Later Enquiries expanded on this, with requirements for close integration between regional MBUs and local specialist perinatal mental health community teams, and for community teams to be adequately resourced to provide senior clinical assessment and appropriate management of all women requiring secondary care.

The last piece of the jigsaw of service organisation fell into place in the 2009–13 Report, which recommended the establishment of perinatal mental health regional networks to coordinate care provision.

As specialist services have expanded rapidly throughout the UK and Ireland over the past 5–10 years, new lessons are emerging on how community peri-natal mental health teams and MBUs should function. The 2017–19 Report highlighted four areas of concern including (i) failure to refer to specialist services; (ii) restrictive referral criteria acting as a block to appropriate care; and (iii) response times from services not taking into account the need for prompt action during and after pregnancy. The fourth concern was the increasingly complex landscape of specialist, enhanced and universal services surrounding the woman and her infant, which was causing confusion and a need to develop clear pathways into care.

The Report reiterated the need for specialist services to have the capacity to assess and manage the care of any woman who met the criteria for general adult mental health services – and to adjust for the altered (usually lower) thresholds for assessment in the perinatal period. Rapid intervention may be necessary given the time constraints imposed by pregnancy and childbirth and the importance of the mother-infant relationship to early child development. Pathways into care must be clear to women and referrers, despite the more complex range of provision (Figure 12.2). It would be ironic if the development of specialist services, long heralded as bringing clarity by acting as a 'one-stop shop' for referrers, became a victim of its own success through its increasing diversity of provision.

Education and training

From the 2000–2 Report onwards, the Enquiries have repeatedly recommended better training in perinatal mental health for both specialists and generalists. These include the need to include perinatal mental health in medical and midwifery curricula and in continuing professional development. With the increasing subspecialisation of adult mental health services, a particular mes-sage arose in the 2009–13 Report around the need for liaison, crisis and home treatment teams to have specific training in the distinctive symptom profile,

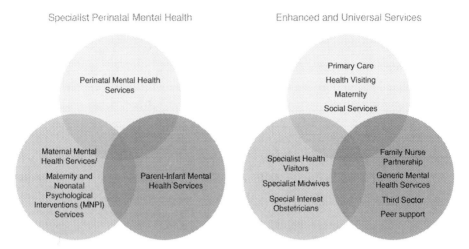

Figure 12.2 Developments in perinatal and infant mental health care provision in the UK

progression and risk management of perinatal mental illness. Concerns of a similar nature arose in the 2017–19 Report.

Substance misuse

Mental health reports in the Enquiries have always sought to learn lessons from the stories of women who died in relation to substance misuse. Again, there are lessons both for individual care and for service organisation. The Enquiries have seen many examples of discontinuity of care, including disengagement and loss to follow-up, often reflecting the complex adversity faced by women with substance misuse and the need for assertive attempts at engagement. A particular point of risk is loss or threatened loss through child protection proceedings. After such events women are at elevated risk of accidental or intentional overdose of illicit drugs.

At an organisational level, most of the women who died were managed by universal services or by enhanced care maternity services. Few were seen by specialist addictions services. Universal services tended to rely on women's accounts of their drug use, often not backed up by independent monitoring. The Enquiries have repeatedly recommended that substance-misusing women should be managed by integrated, multidisciplinary specialist services nested within maternity services and that monitoring should include drug assay and/ or independent measures of alcohol use.

A new lesson from the 2017–19 Enquiry recognised the additional vulnerability to relapse in the postnatal period. It recommended that, even where women had shown improvement in their substance use in pregnancy, they should be reassessed in the early postpartum period if they had contact with addictions services before or during pregnancy.

Women discussed but not counted in Mental Health Reports

A small but important group of women die from a range of underlying physical conditions where their care is adversely influenced by misattribution of symptoms to mental ill health. The 2006–8 Report highlighted examples of women with conditions as diverse as tuberculosis, eclampsia and subarachnoid haemorrhage, whose symptoms were varyingly ascribed to anorexia nervosa, anxiety or depression, thus delaying appropriate care. The Report provided guidance ('Back to Basics') which identified where clinicians should exercise caution in diagnosing mental illness in the absence of clear indication (Figure 12.3).

A further group of women, frequently discussed in the mental health reports, are those who die by homicide. This group, like those with substance

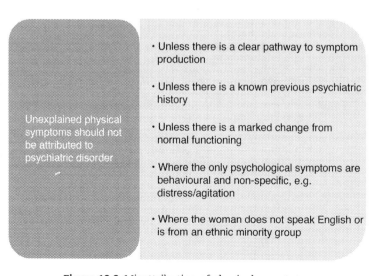

Figure 12.3 Misattribution of physical symptoms

misuse, frequently experienced multiple adversity, including adverse early life experiences and domestic abuse. The need for proactive, assertive engagement was again a recurrent message.

How the Enquiries have changed service provision

In 1991, shortly before the first Report making specific mental health recommendations, the *British Medical Journal* published a survey of the care of women with puerperal psychiatric disorders in England and Wales. The authors, Prettyman and Friedman, identified 133 mother and baby beds but found that almost half of all districts admitted the women to general adult facilities and 1 in 10 had no provision for joint admission either to an MBU or to a general ward. Just under half of the identified MBUs consisted of one or two beds, making it highly unlikely that they were able to provide specialist care.

Thirty years later the picture had changed. As of 2021 there were 22 MBUs across England, Scotland and Wales, with a total of 169 beds, but, more importantly, all were in units with an average of 6–8 beds and with specialist staff caring for women and infants.

Although it is more difficult to quantify the change in community provision, there has been an exponential rise in specialist teams across the UK. In 2014, eight community services were inaugural members of the Royal College of Psychiatrists' Perinatal Quality Network for Community Services. By 2021 that number had risen to more than 70.

While these developments cannot all be ascribed to the Enquiries, their influence on individual practice and on the fostering of evidence-based guidance has been profound. Specialist guidance from the National Institute for Health and Care Excellence and the Scottish Intercollegiate Guideline Network (SIGN) cites the Enquiries in relation to recommendations on clinical care and service development, and has strongly influenced the standards set out in National Health Service and governmental guidance and developed by the Royal College of Psychiatrists' Perinatal Quality Network. These standards have been widely adopted by commissioners and services throughout the UK. The tier of managed clinical network provision, now almost universal at the regional or national levels in the UK, was also presaged by a recommendation in the 2009–13 Report from the Enquiry.

Conclusion

The Confidential Enquiries have had a lasting effect on the development and quality of perinatal mental health services in the UK and Ireland and on the care women receive. Their methodology has seeded new reporting structures across the globe, widening their influence. It has been encouraging to see a number of international reports which now include deaths due to psychiatric causes, extending to the end of the first postnatal year, in countries such as France and Switzerland and in regions of the USA. In the future this will allow improved learning across nations and cultures, helping to reduce stigma and promote parity with physical health.

There is a further important if paradoxical lesson for all mental health professionals and services in general. Many of the Enquiries' recommendations stem from the distinctive presentations and risks associated with perinatal mental illness, and the service responses required to meet those specific needs. It is striking, however, that lessons learned often derive from therapeutic contact that has *not* met some core features of good clinical care.

These include taking a comprehensive history, listening carefully, paying attention not only to what the woman says, but to all aspects of her mental state, and hearing the concerns of relatives. In formulating management plans, the lessons include recognising that risk is dynamic, that symptoms evolve and that the woman should be assessed as an individual, not bound by diagnostic preconceptions or service constraints.

If these lessons can be brought to the attention of all mental health professionals and organisations, the Enquiries will have achieved something far beyond their core duty to improve the care of childbearing women, their infants and their families.

13 THE MOTHERS WHO DIED: SOCIAL DETERMINANTS OF MATERNAL HEALTH

Before the early twentieth century death in childbirth was both common and undiscriminating. From the impoverished mothers in the workhouses of Victorian England, through those who worked in fields, factories or shops, to the comfortable well-to-do and even the aristocracy, all women were at risk of the big maternal killers of the time such as infection, bleeding and toxaemia (high blood pressure of pregnancy and eclampsia).

The development of modern obstetrics and midwifery and the introduction of legal abortion markedly changed this. The tide of deaths from these Direct obstetric conditions, which can only occur in pregnancy, has receded and now most mothers die from Indirect causes. These are usually pre-existing medical or mental health conditions which, although not directly due to pregnancy, are adversely affected by the changes pregnancy brings. Thus conditions such as heart disease, epilepsy and psychiatric ill health account for much larger proportions of maternal deaths than they used to. And these Indirect deaths are also far commoner in women with underlying physical or mental health issues and who may be socially vulnerable in other ways.

The social factors

Adverse social factors which can affect pregnancy include poverty, deprivation, minority ethnicity, limited English language and refugee status. Lifestyle factors such as drug and alcohol misuse, poor nutrition and obesity also have harmful effects. Mothers and their babies are also severely affected by domestic abuse or by people around them who limit their autonomy and control their access to care. Examples of this include trafficked women, 'mail-order' or underage brides and women living with the effects of genital mutilation or cutting.

These findings pose the question of how such avoidable inequities can be identified, reduced and eventually eliminated. It is well known that apart from receiving high-quality clinical care, key determinants of maternal well-being are care early in pregnancy and regular check-ups. Efforts have been made to make services more accessible, but much of what is needed to address the underlying issues lies far beyond the scope of the health services. This problem needs to be addressed through coherent, coordinated action by national and local government departments, agencies and stakeholders.

Victorian attitudes to women's health

Inequalities in women's health have existed for centuries. Deaths in pregnancy, one of the greatest killers of young women, tended to be overlooked and regarded almost as an occupational hazard, while studies of men's health have a long history. In the 1830s Edwin Chadwick, whom some regard as the father of modern public health, found a 15-year difference in life expectancy between better-off men and those of working age in the poorer parts of London, and showed that this was due to overcrowding, poor sanitation and infection. His work eventually led to the 1848 Public Health Act with legislation for street cleaning, sewage and clean water. His plea for indoor toilets, however, was not heard until after the Second World War.

Even though deaths in childbirth were still shockingly common, and despite the growing interest in health inequalities, the focus in the first part of the nineteenth century remained resolutely on variations in death rates among men. It took a woman to change this. Once she returned from the Crimea, Florence Nightingale turned her pioneering statistical gaze on the number of deaths among women giving birth in workhouses and the charitable 'lying-in' hospitals (Figure 13.1). Better-off mothers tended to give birth in the relative comfort of their own homes, attended by a physician or obstetrician. In 1872 Nightingale calculated that 'for every 2 women who died delivered at home, 15 must have died if delivered in a lying-in hospital'.

The deaths were mostly due to sepsis, which spread rapidly in public facilities due to poor hygiene. Deprivation, poverty, the stigma of illegitimacy and other adverse life circumstances had led these women to deliver in such places. But Florence Nightingale was aware that mothers at home were also at high risk of dying, and she also asked, 'why is it that, at home, 1 out of every 128 must die? If the facts are correct, then one cannot help feeling that they present a very strong prima facie case for inquiring, with the view of devising a remedy for such a state of things.' She would have welcomed the advent of the Confidential Enquiries into Maternal Deaths (CEMDs).

Fact-finding begins

By the start of the twentieth century the high maternal mortality rate had at last become a matter of major public and professional concern. The highest death

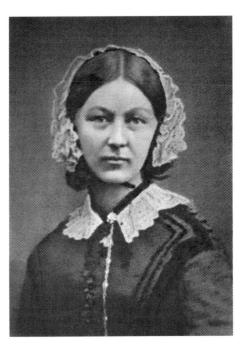

Figure 13.1 Florence Nightingale (1820–1910) argued for major reforms and professional training for all staff caring for the 'sick poor' and is regarded as the founder of modern nursing and midwifery practice. However, not everyone was enthusiastic and many members of the medical profession were hostile to her ideas. A number of anonymous doctors writing in the *British Medical Journal* accused her of 'having a kind, womanly heart', 'sublime simplicity' and being 'purely sentimental'.

rates in the country, in Rochdale, outnumbered London rates by nearly 10 to 1. Initially it was suggested that this difference was due to the effects of malnutrition or the poor working environments in the mills. In 1929, however, a detailed confidential enquiry, the first of its kind, showed the main factors to be a lack of antenatal care, limited healthcare knowledge in the general population and poor clinical care. The action taken on these findings led to a dramatic decline in the local death rate within five years, the first real example of evidence-based improvements in maternal care. It laid the path for similar enquires to start elsewhere, ultimately resulting in the national Confidential Enquiry in 1952 (see Chapter 2).

During the 1930s national reports on maternal mortality started to include short paragraphs on the wider social circumstances of the mothers who died. This was an achievement in itself because data collection systems were in their infancy, the National Health Service (NHS) did not yet exist and it was only possible to collect basic information such as a mother's age, marital status and perhaps her previous pregnancies. Nonetheless, all of these reports identified that, when compared to southern England, maternal death rates were three times higher in South Wales, the 'Black' country of the manufacturing Midlands and some industrial cities of the north.

The urban mothers who died tended to have been poor, lived in overcrowded tenements and depended on charitable and highly stretched health services, whereas those in rural areas faced an almost entire lack of maternity services. In one report mention was made of 'racial' differences between these areas, but data on ethnic groups were not collected so presumably this related to other social characteristics of the women.

The reports of the 1930s also first described the variation in the availability of antenatal or hospital-based obstetric facilities within a reasonable distance of the mother's home, this being a crucial determinant of health – although sometimes in unexpected ways. One author blamed the high rural maternal death rate on 'the building of hundreds of little cottage hospitals' where low-quality caesarean sections were performed by staff with little obstetric expertise.

The early Enquiries, 1952–1994

In 1952, when the Confidential Enquiries started in England and Wales, statistics showed that, infection aside, mothers still died more frequently in Wales than in England, and that, within England. maternal mortality rates remained higher in rural areas. Apart from this the reports that covered the first 40 years of the Enquiry (which by 1994 had grown to include Scotland and Northern Ireland) contained virtually no information about the social circumstances of the mothers who died. Age and the number of previous pregnancies were the only indicators routinely available, and it was already known that older and more parous mothers were at higher risk of complications and death.

The first CEMD Report, for 1952–4, did attempt to use marital status and wealth (presumably guessed at by the assessors) as indicators for the mothers who died from abortion, but not for deaths from other causes. Successive reports contained only tables on marital status, presumably as a proxy for some form of social characteristic, but all this showed was an increase in births outside marriage over the following years. The report for 1988–90 eventually concluded that 'being unmarried was not a risk factor for maternal mortality overall'. This has remained so ever since.

The Black Report and the resurgence of the public health movement

By the 1970s it was becoming clear that it was untenable to assume that the NHS, left to its own devices, would eventually eliminate health inequalities. The resurgence of interest in and expanding literature on inequities and their links to the social determinants of health led, in 1977, to the Labour government asking Sir Douglas Black, an eminent professor of medicine and ex-president of the Royal College of Physicians, to chair an enquiry into this.

His report showed what many had suspected: not only did the poorest people still have the highest rates of ill health and death, but the gap was widening. Although the 'Black Report' considered maternal deaths only in passing because the numbers were relatively small, it found that rates were at least doubled in women of the lowest occupational group, unskilled workers, compared to the professional classes (Figure 13.2).

The Black Report's publication in 1980 was essentially suppressed by the Conservative government. Only 260 photocopies were ever made available – to selected media contacts on a bank holiday Monday. But far from the facts being suppressed, the touch paper was lit. The authors held their own press conferences, after which there was a public outcry followed by a rapid resurgence of the public health movement and advocacy for 'health for all'.

But nothing was actually done for another 10 years, when inequalities became the subject of other nationally commissioned reports, notably by Sir Donald Acheson and also *The Health of the Nation*, a government report published in 1992 as a response to the World Health Organization's (WHO) *Global Strategy for Health for All by the Year 2000*. Presumably for lack of data, none of these UK reports looked at differences in health outcomes by ethnicity. Nonetheless they all came to the same conclusion: inequalities could not be ignored or wished away.

1990: A question mark over the need for the Enquiries

During the first 40 years of the Confidential Enquiries, inequalities were barely mentioned, even following the Black Report. The great successes of the CEMD's early years were largely due to improvements in clinical care and legislation for safe, legal abortion. Through the development and implementation of clinical guidelines and other improvements, by the early 1990s the United Kingdom had arguably one of the lowest maternal death rates in the world. As a result, within the government and among other commentators, questions were being asked about why the Enquiries should continue. After all, it was

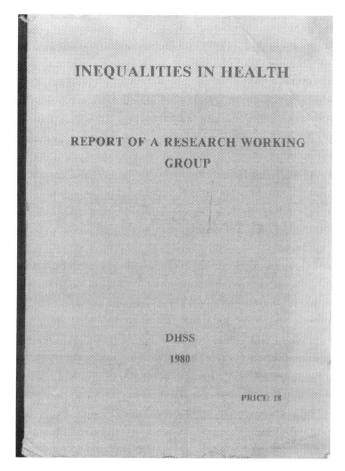

Figure 13.2 The Black Report (1980). In its foreword Secretary of State for Social Services Patrick Jenkin stated, 'It will be seen that the Group has reached the view that the causes of health inequalities are so deep rooted that only a major and wide-ranging programme of public expenditure is capable of altering the pattern. I must make it clear that additional expenditure … is quite unrealistic in present or any foreseeable economic circumstances, quite apart from any judgement that may be formed of the effectiveness of such expenditure in dealing with the problems identified.'

argued, the number of women dying from pregnancy-related causes had probably reached 'an irreducible minimum'.

This thinking has proven seriously mistaken, partly in its dismissal of the prospects of further advances in clinical care, but also in ignoring growing public concerns about equity and the possible social determinants of poor maternal health. Fortunately, enlightened Department of Health officials eventually decided not only to save the Enquiry but to extend its scope and appointed a public health physician as the Department of Health's new director, with an expanded assessment panel and an editorial group composed of the most respected professionals.

A new kind of Report: Why Mothers Die, 1994–1996

While continuing with the existing agenda, the first revised Report, for 1994–6, was expanded to cover (as best it could, for the data were still poor) the part played by the mothers' social circumstances (Figure 13.3). Many women whose deaths had been described in the earlier reports also had coexisting medical and mental health conditions, and it had been noticed that a significant number had been obese. The new-style Report provided more in-depth

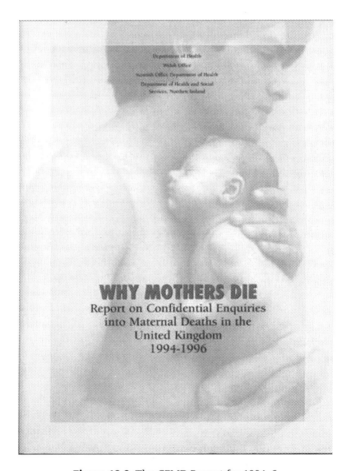

Figure 13.3 The CEMD Report for 1994–6

analysis of these and other such factors, and findings in these areas have become essential reading in successive publications.

The Report's presentation also changed. Gone were the uninviting covers of the past and in came an arresting yet simple title – *Why Mothers Die* – and pictures to engage readers' attention. In subsequent editions the name was changed again to *Saving Mothers Lives*, to signal that the purpose was not just to list the numbers and types of deaths, but also to learn lessons and stimulate improvement of care. By 2016–18 it had become *Saving Lives, Improving Mothers' Care*.

But *Why Mothers Die* represented more than a change in name and an extension of scope. It was also a marked change in philosophy, from an outdated medical model to one that recognised women as individuals who had died before their time. They were no longer described as numbers, people or cases, and the statistics became humanised; they became women and mothers. The assessors then went 'beyond the numbers', which was the name of the seminal WHO programme that arose from this enquiry. It recognised that for each dying mother there was a story to be told, that those stories held clues as why they had died, and that these in turn could indicate what could be done to improve future outcomes.

'Ignorant or self-neglectful mothers'

One regrettable feature of the early Reports was a tendency to blame the mother for her death. Failures to seek antenatal care or to comply with treatment were commonly cited. This was an easy out for health professionals who wished to avoid scrutiny, and their state of denial prevented both individual learning and wider improvements in clinical standards. In one early Report, in the 1950s, women were blamed for more than a quarter of the 406 deaths which were considered avoidable and 'only a few of these uncooperative patients were of low or disordered mentality'.

But while women themselves were often blamed because of 'their refusal or neglect to follow medical advice or to seek such advice', there was a growing recognition that for many women their social circumstances were such that seeking maternity care was low on their list of priorities. To this end the Report also says: 'some degree of responsibility rests with the doctors and midwives to gain the confidence of ignorant or self-neglectful mothers, to study their problems and to help them despite themselves'.

From 1994 onwards, instead of treating mothers as in some way complicit, the focus changed to trying to understand the barriers to care each woman faced. New questions in the assessment included: 'What could have been done differently to help this mother?' 'What could professionals, health service managers and policy planners have done better?' 'What can be done to meet their needs in future?'

Accessing and keeping in touch with care

As today, over the past years of the Reports many of the mothers who died were vulnerable and lived with multiple and complex problems – what the latest Report for 2016–18 refers to as 'a constellation of systemic biases (Figure 13.4) (see Chapter 14). These often made it difficult for them to seek or maintain contact with maternity or other services.

In the 2006–8 CEMD Report, 44% of substance-abusing women or those known to child protection services did not register early enough in pregnancy or regularly failed to attend for antenatal care. This was also the case for 33% of the mothers who reported domestic abuse. A quarter of mothers from the most deprived areas also found it hard to attend. The very latest findings show that, in 2016–18, nearly 30% of the mothers who died still did not receive the recommended level of care.

Deprivation and socio-economic characteristics

Since 2004 it has been possible to link the mother's home postcode to a national deprivation score calculated from multiple indicators of deprivation, including employment, education and environmental factors. Each postcode falls into one of five deprivation categories. As expected, there is an excess risk of maternal death for mothers living in the more deprived areas. In 2003–5 the rate in the most deprived group was five times greater than in the least deprived. In 2016–18 this had dropped to a threefold excess risk, but the difference was still statistically significant.

Another indicator of social circumstances is the National Statistics Socio-Economic Classification (NS-SEC) code which recorded the occupation of the mother's partner, or in the case of a single woman, her own occupation. When first calculated in 2003–5, the rates of death for women with unemployed partners were seven times higher than for those who had a partner in employment and four times higher for unemployed single mothers compared those in work. Perhaps because of the advent of more locally accessible services, the risk seems to have dropped to two to three times higher for unemployed mothers today.

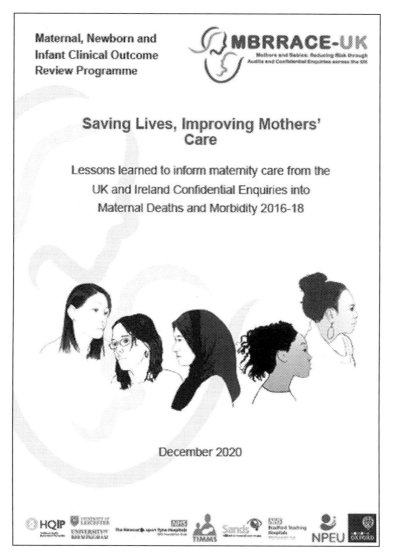

Figure 13.4 The MBRRACE-UK Report for 2016–18

Ethnicity

Hard as it is to believe today, none of the great public health reports of the later twentieth century addressed differences in health outcomes by ethnicity. One explanation is the lack of data. The earlier CEMD Reports also fell short in this respect because, apart from country of birth, official and comprehensive data indicating ethnicity for England, Wales and Scotland were not routinely collected until the 1991 census. Collection of data on ethnic groups had been planned 10 years earlier, in the 1981 census, but representatives of these groups resisted, as they considered the collection of such information discriminatory.

Information about the ethnic groups of NHS patients, including mothers, was not routinely collected until the Hospital Episode Statistics system was introduced in 1995, and even then the data varied in completeness and quality for many years.

Eventually it was possible for the newly revamped Report for 94–6 to start to identify the ethnic groups of the mothers who died. According to the best estimates at the time, Black mothers overall (a composite of women of African, Caribbean or 'other' Black heritage, as it was then described) were three times more likely to die than White mothers.

Gradually data collection improved. Coverage was still only 67% in the 2000–2 Report, but with judicious analysis allowing more accurate estimates of death rates by ethnic group, even larger discrepancies were revealed. Black African mothers, including substantial proportions of refugees and asylum-seeking women, were at seven times the risk of maternal death compared to White women, and Black Caribbean mothers were at three times the risk.

The difference in rates dropped from sevenfold to an average of fourfold in all successive reports. Rather than stubbornly remaining the same, however, the gap has recently widened. The latest Report, for 2016–18, revealed a death rate for Black women that was five times higher than that of White women. A twofold increase in risk was reported for women who identified as Asian or from mixed ethnic backgrounds, and this has remained remarkably consistent since data collection began (see Figure 13.5).

Among the many recent initiatives that have emerged since these findings were the development of the Race Equality Taskforce and the first Black Women's Maternal Health Awareness Week. Guidance is still being developed by professional organisations for obstetricians, midwives and other stakeholders.

The NHS response: a raft of initiatives, policies and publications

These initiatives are very welcome but overall change has been a long time coming. The first real national policy response to the inequalities exposed in the hard-hitting CEMD Reports of the early 2000s was led by the Department of Health for England, which, in 2008, published *Maternity Matters* and the accompanying *National Service Framework* (Figure 13.6). Similar policies were developed by the other home countries. The aim was to promote 'choice, access

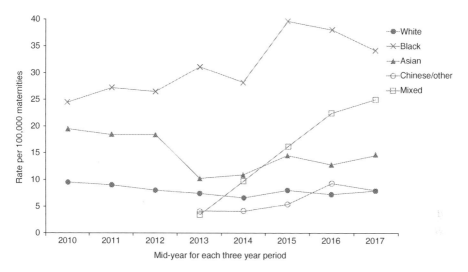

Figure 13.5 Maternal mortality rates, 2009–18, among women from ethnic groups in the UK (from *Saving Lives, Improving Mothers' Care*, 2016–18)

and continuity of care in a safe service' with the vision of 'flexible services with a focus on the needs of the individual, especially those who are more vulnerable or disadvantaged'.

It also promoted individualised maternity care plans with a named midwife, one-to-one care in labour and midwife-led antenatal care in the community or by the 'maternity team'. It was expected that care for women with complex social needs should 'be provided in partnership with other agencies' such as children's services, domestic abuse teams, substance misuse services, drug and alcohol teams'.

Much in the provision of NHS maternity services changed for the better as a result of *Maternity Matters* but this appears to have had little impact on adverse maternal health outcomes. Inequalities remained among the small number of mothers who died, and research on mothers who survived severe complications of pregnancy found similar factors which give them also the same excess risk of severe complications as those who died.

In 2016 another policy drive, NHS England's *Better Births: Five Year Forward Plan*, sought to improve maternity outcomes with by-now-familiar means: more personalised services, continuity of care with a known midwife, closer linkages with mental health services, multidisciplinary and cross-boundary working and improved quality of care (Figure 13.7). However, *Better Births* did not really address the inequalities agenda and it rather dismissed maternal

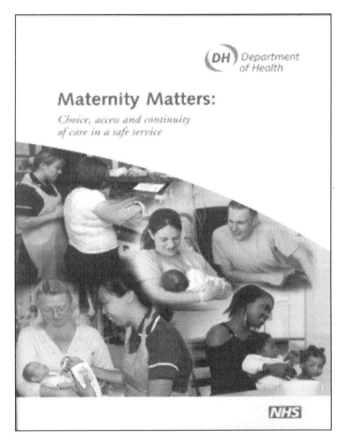

Figure 13.6 2008: The national framework for maternity services promoted the local delivery of high-quality, safe and accessible services that are women-focussed and family-centred. Services should be accessible to all women and be designed to take account of their individual needs.

mortality in general because the overall rates had declined a little over the previous10 years. It failed to acknowledge that, while the overall numbers may have fallen, the inequities between those mothers who died had not.

Better Births was rapidly followed by its implementation plan, the *Maternity Transformation Programme*. Among other things, services were encouraged 'to engage better with diverse communities'. Even more recently the stark findings of the 2016–18 *Saving Lives* report resulted in a target being set in the 2019 *NHS Long-Term Plan for England*: 'At least 75% of women from Black and ethnic minority communities and those from the most deprived groups should have continuity of care from their midwife throughout pregnancy' (Figure 13.8).

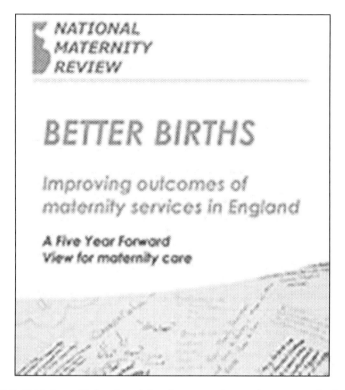

Figure 13.7 2016: *Better Births.* Our vision for maternity services across England is for them to become safer, more personalised, kinder, professional and more family friendly, where every woman has access to information to enable her to make decisions about her care, and where she and her baby can access support centred around their individual needs and circumstances.

The *Better Births* report sets an ambitious target to halve deaths among pregnant women by 50% by 2025. It also seeks to halve stillbirths and deaths in newborn babies, whose own outcomes are greatly affected by their mothers' underlying health status. While these objectives are laudable, they are laughable. They demonstrate the disconnect between lofty policy declarations and the reality on the ground.

They fail to address or even recognise the abundance of evidence reviewed briefly here, and available in far more breadth and depth elsewhere, that maternal health and well-being are not uniquely dependent on the health services but are severely compromised by the multitude of long-standing underlying factors that cannot be turned off like a switch.

Deprivation, vulnerability and ethnicity aside, successive generations of women will need support to take control over their lives so they value

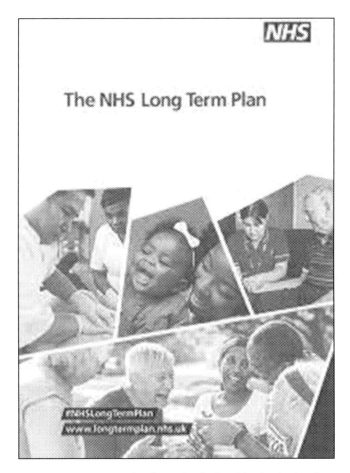

Figure 13.8 2019: *NHS Long-Term Plan for England.* The objective is that, by 2024, 75% of women from Black and minority ethnic communities and a similar percentage of women from the most deprived groups will receive continuity of care from their midwife throughout pregnancy, labour and the postnatal period. The aim is to reduce the disparities in maternal and perinatal mortality.

themselves more by becoming physically and mentally healthier. Addressing these wider factors effectively – and to the extent suggested by these impossible targets – lies far beyond the scope of health systems alone.

Conclusions

Since the beginning of the discussions about inequity and vulnerability in the 1994–6 Report, and despite the many policy initiatives, reforms, reports, working groups and focus discussions, little seems to have changed. In fact the challenges seem even greater and disparities and gaps are widening. To bring this message home all one needs to do is consider the latest figures for 2016–18. They show that 90% of the 510 mothers who died during pregnancy or up to one year after birth were, in some measure, socially vulnerable. And three-quarters of them had pre-existing medical or mental health conditions.

Such findings are not new. In the 1930s Sir Henry Brackenbury, a distinguished doctor of the day, when commenting on the high maternal death rate, presciently said: 'I cannot help suspecting that, however important administrative and clinical factors may be, the main explanation may yet be found in those biological, physical, dietetic, sociological and even psychological factors which so far appear to have received insufficient attention.' Surely the same must be said 90 years later.

14 THE LEGACY IN THE UNITED KINGDOM: THE CONCEPT OF 'NEAR MISS' AND THE NEED TO KEEP SAVING LIVES

From 1952 until 2011, when the last triennial Report was published, the Confidential Enquiries into Maternal Deaths (CEMDs) were directed by a Principal Medical Officer in the Department of Health. After 1999, however, the links between the Department and the Enquiries were weakened by repeated reorganisations. The Confidential Enquiry into Maternal and Child Health (CEMACH) was followed by the Centre for Maternal and Child Enquiries (CMACE) (see Chapter 3) and a more fundamental change came in 2012. Following a competitive tendering process, the Enquiry moved to its present home, the National Perinatal Epidemiology Unit (NPEU) in the University of Oxford.

The NPEU is a multidisciplinary research unit established in 1978 after a joint request for such a unit from the Royal College of Obstetricians and Gynaecologists (RCOG) and the British Paediatric Association. Its first director was Sir Iain Chalmers. When the CEMD moved there in 2012 it became part of a new body with a new acronym, MBRRACE-UK (Mothers and Babies: Reducing Risk through Audits and Confidential Enquiries in the UK). Since its foundation MBRRACE-UK CEMD has been directed by Professor Marian Knight.

MBRRACE-UK

A new era had begun for the CEMD, bringing the opportunity to implement fresh ideas, and some which had previously seemed impossible to put into practice. Within the specification for the Enquiries were two key changes: a requirement for annual reporting and the addition of topic-based enquiries into 'near-misses'. A 'near-miss' has been defined as a 'severe life-threatening obstetric complication necessitating urgent medical intervention in order to prevent likely death of the mother'.

The change to annual reporting recognised the need for more timely publication of findings and recommendations to maintain the continuous improvement in the quality of care underpinned by the Enquiry. The inclusion of 'near-miss' enquiries was a recognition not only of the success of the Enquiry in reducing maternal deaths to low numbers – almost abolishing, for instance, maternal deaths from anaesthetic causes (see Chapter 11) – but also of the need for better understanding of the long-lasting and potentially life-changing impacts of pregnancy complications in women who survive them.

Alongside these new developments the methodology of the Enquiry evolved. This was prompted by the need for speed to produce annual reports, by advancements in information technology and by recognition of the insecure nature of postal transfer of medical records. A substantial decrease in the funding provided for the Enquiry also underpinned the move to a single-tier system whereby the regional offices were abolished with the closure of CMACE and a single tier of national assessors was established.

In keeping with the changing patterns of maternal deaths and continuing recognition of the central role of midwifery in modern childbirth care, new specialist assessors in cardiology, neurology and infectious diseases were introduced to the Enquiry, along with a substantially expanded cadre of midwifery assessors.

Assessment of the care women received was undertaken through an online platform specifically developed to view anonymised medical records. Simultaneous review of each woman's records by between 10 and 15 specialist assessors considerably sped up the review process, countering the criticism of the length of time required to generate CEMD recommendations. The added value of multidisciplinary discussion was maintained by panel writing meetings at which all reviews were discussed by a group including members from all relevant professional disciplines to draw together the key lessons to improve care.

Near-misses and the United Kingdom Obstetric Surveillance System (UKOSS)

It is estimated that, for every woman who dies during or after pregnancy in the UK, around 100 experience a life-threatening complication. Thus, in the early 2020s when around 1 in 10,000 pregnant or post-partum women died, around 1 in every 100 had a near-miss where they almost died. Conducting enquiries into the care these women received could therefore provide more widespread lessons for improving care and preventing not only mortality, but also severe morbidity.

While not a problem in the UK, where the history of the CEMD as detailed in these pages has led to widespread trust and understanding of its purpose and benefits, in many countries reviews of maternal deaths are perceived as threatening. Confidential Enquiries into near-misses, also known as 'great saves' in the South African CEMD, may be seen as less threatening by individual doctors, midwives and hospitals. Examining near-misses can thus provide a way of introducing Confidential Enquiries in countries which do not have the UK's historical precedent for mortality reviews.

The transition of the CEMD to the MBRRACE-UK collaboration was helped by the fact that the United Kingdom Obstetric Surveillance System (UKOSS) had been established at the NPEU in 2005. The UKOSS is a national research platform for the study of uncommon severe pregnancy complications. It involves all obstetric units in the UK in routine notification of such events to the NPEU. Linking the two systems allowed comprehensive epidemiological research into near-miss complications through the UKOSS to be complemented by in-depth review, through the CEMD, of the quality of care given to individual women.

The added value of the CEMM

For the new Confidential Enquiry into Maternal Morbidity (CEMM), life-threatening events had to be identified. This was done in different ways according to the topic being studied – for example, an existing UKOSS study was used to identify pulmonary embolism in pregnancy and immediately post-partum. Following notification of the event, the Enquiry methodology for the CEMM remained exactly the same as for the CEMD. Linking the CEMM with the other parts of MBRRACE's work brought added value to the Enquiries. The following examples come from three important conditions – haemorrhage, breast cancer and psychosis.

Haemorrhage

The 2013–15 CEMD highlighted a near doubling of the rate of maternal death from obstetric haemorrhage in the UK. This worrying rise was almost entirely due to bleeding following abnormal placental adherence caused by invasion of placental tissue into and through the muscle of the womb – a condition associated with previous caesarean birth. The increase was therefore perhaps symptomatic of changing childbirth trends towards more intervention.

This illustrates one of the important reasons for maintaining the CEMD even when maternal deaths are relatively uncommon. Trends and patterns are continually changing – in the population of women who give birth, in clinical practice and in the policy environment. These changes can impact maternal mortality and rapid action is essential to maintain the safety of childbirth. In this example, the CEMD recognised that several of the women who died were already known to have an abnormally adherent placenta and had had repeated previous episodes of bleeding, but were cared for at home. The clear recommendation was that in future such women should be cared for in hospital, where facilities are immediately available to respond to catastrophic bleeding.

The CEMM added important observations to this message. Its next report, published in 2018, identified several women who had clear risk factors for an abnormally adherent placenta which were not identified or acted on. As a result, their severe bleeding at the time of childbirth was unanticipated and required life-changing interventions such as hysterectomy. These might have been prevented if their risk had been recognised.

Furthermore, deaths from traumatic bleeding were rare in the CEMD but in contrast the CEMM found that a significant number of women had unrecognised bleeding due to uterine and vaginal tears at the time of childbirth. The Enquiry emphasised the importance of monitoring to obtain early warning of such bleeding to prevent the need for interventions such as hysterectomy or blood transfusion. These examples clearly illustrate the additional benefits for women's long-term health of the CEMM approach.

New constraints

Nevertheless, a worrying development arose during the process of approving the 2018 Report for publication. Changes to government, to NHS structures and to legal frameworks over the lifetime of the CEMD have altered not only the organisation responsible for delivering the Enquiry, but also the funding organisation. With this came additional layers of bureaucracy. Before the findings can be published, approval is required from several organisations, with detailed revisions to the content of any publication in a three-stage process.

The Enquiry has always touted itself as an independent assessment of where improvements to UK maternity care need to be made, and it has not held back from stating truth to power, even when this is uncomfortable. The 2018 Report had, in several places but notably in reference to the findings concerning haemorrhage, used a framework first described in a 2016 *Lancet* series on maternal health. That series highlighted the themes of 'too much too soon' and 'too little too late', representing the extremes of maternity care which need to be addressed to improve maternal health globally. When the report was revised for publication the authors were required to remove several references to these themes. This maybe reduced discomfort to the reader but suggested a disturbing move towards removal of independent editorial control.

Allied to this threat to editorial independence have been requirements from the funding organisation which could limit the future impact of both the CEMD and the CEMM. All Reports are required to have no more than 5–10 recommendations, and recommendations should be cost-neutral. While most messages from the Enquiry now reference existing guidance on clinical care, as evidenced, for example, by Chapter 7 on hypertension management, the Enquiry has played an important role in driving the development of guidance where none exists, and this is an aspect which will need careful safeguarding.

Most perplexingly perhaps, the Enquiry team is now prevented from liaising with the media in advance of issuing of a report. This seriously weakens the Enquiries' impact. Chapter 2 described how the local media played a vital role in the success of the Rochdale Experiment in 1930, and Chapter 3 pointed out that the launch of each CEMD Report in the early 2000s was a media event which caught the attention of women and professionals. The new embargo on press releases removes the ability of the Enquiries to empower women by using the media to disseminate messages to improve their care.

Breast cancer

A recurring message over many years of CEMD reports is that pregnant and post-partum women should be treated in the same way as non-pregnant people unless there is a clear reason not to do so. Nonetheless numerous examples exist of potentially beneficial investigations or treatment being withheld from pregnant and breastfeeding women for inappropriate reasons. As noted in Chapter 10, these may be misplaced concerns about fetal risk, a lack of recognition of the benefits of treatment to the woman herself or a simple lack of expertise and experience in pregnancy medicine.

Women make reproductive health decisions in the context of cumulative anxiety-provoking messages which associate risk with almost any food, drink, medication or underlying health condition (see Figure 14.1). Clinicians are subject to the same influences, potentially increasing their focus on pregnancy concerns to the detriment of women's health. Multiple reports have noted that pregnant and post-partum women's diagnoses were delayed because X-rays or similar investigations were not carried out, and the 2015 MBRRACE Report noted the same for women with cancer.

The 2015 Report also highlighted the finding that treatments such as chemotherapy or radiotherapy were inappropriately withheld because women were pregnant at the time of cancer diagnosis. Consequently women

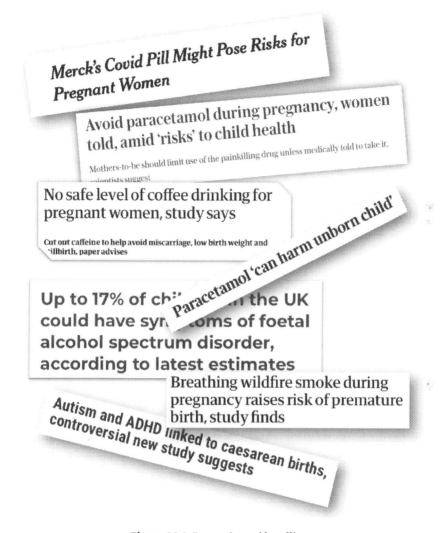

Figure 14.1 Recent 'scare' headlines

became severely unwell, necessitating an unplanned premature birth, or a preterm birth was planned to allow treatment to begin. The Report emphasised that chemotherapy can be used in pregnancy and that iatrogenic preterm birth has long-term consequences for infant health and development. It was reassuring that three years later the Enquiry found that delayed chemotherapy and unnecessary premature births in women with cancer were rarely evident.

The CEMM identified that, in women with breast cancer, inappropriately withholding investigations not only led to delays in diagnosis, but also meant that the stage of the woman's disease was not fully assessed. As a result, several women underwent extensive operative treatments which were unnecessary for their stage of disease. Full staging investigations would have prevented these operations, with their attendant risks, being undertaken during pregnancy.

Psychosis

Addressing maternal mental as well as physical health has become a priority for the CEMD (see Chapter 12). Recommendations have focussed on forward planning (Figure 14.2) with early identification of risk, timely response by mental health services, availability of care in a mother and baby unit and discussion and planning for future pregnancies after an episode of pregnancy-associated psychosis.

In 2017 the CEMM reported an investigation into the care of women who had an episode of psychosis during or after a previous pregnancy. There were examples of excellence where women whose care in a previous pregnancy had not been well managed, but they went on to have early intervention in

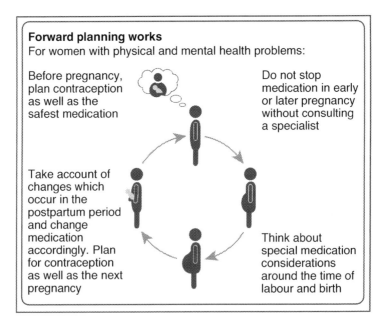

Figure 14.2 Infographic from the 2017 CEMD Report illustrating steps at which forward planning may prevent maternal deaths

a subsequent pregnancy. They were treated to minimise risk, did not relapse acutely and remained safely at home with their families. In this instance the added value of the CEMM lay in clearly illustrating the positive outcomes for both women and their babies when messages for care from the CEMD are implemented.

Continued need for the CEMD

The success of the CEMD has perhaps been its own worst enemy within the UK. It continues to be held up as a global gold standard (see Chapter 15) but, in the UK, where the number of women dying during or up to a year after the end of pregnancy reduced to fewer than 200 per year, the feeling grew within government that women's deaths during or after pregnancy were too few to be worth investigating. Countering this argument became a regular activity. Two examples show the clear need for ongoing enquiries – the case of valproate and the worsening disparities in mortality rates among women from different ethnic groups.

The case of valproate

Sodium valproate is a drug used to treat epilepsy or mental health conditions. During the 2010s evidence crystallised that exposure to valproate during pregnancy could lead to various physical and developmental problems in childhood. Doctors were advised to ensure that, because of these risks, women of reproductive age avoided valproate even if they were not planning pregnancy. The 'Valproate Pregnancy Prevention Programme' was instituted, with very negative and anxiety-provoking language aimed at women. Three years after its introduction, the CEMD identified a significant increase in the number of women dying from 'Sudden Unexpected Death in Epilepsy' (SUDEP). While no women were taking valproate – and thus their fetus was protected – most of the women who died had had uncontrolled seizures before pregnancy, either because they had stopped taking any anti-epileptic medication for fear of its effect in pregnancy, or because the drugs they were taking were ineffective. As a direct consequence of a programme designed to protect the unborn infant, women were dying because their need for effective medication was not recognised or emphasised. As Chapter 10 points out, most had received no specialist epilepsy care in pregnancy.

The valproate story emphasises the need for ongoing surveillance and enquiries into maternal deaths even when they have become uncommon. Well-intentioned policy changes may have adverse consequences that can only be identified – and remedial action planned – through a continuous programme. Similarly, public health emergencies may arise in which rapid learning about the care of women who die during or after pregnancy may have the potential to save many future lives – the COVID-19 pandemic being an obvious example (see later in this chapter).

Black Lives Matter

The CEMD first identified differences in maternal mortality rates between women of different ethnic groups in its Report for 1994–6, published in 1998 (see Chapter 13). The Enquiries continued to document this disparity with little evidence of a major policy response until it became evident, towards the end of the 2010s, that the inequality was widening. Without the work of the Enquiry this widening disparity would otherwise have been masked within an overall static maternal mortality figure.

Three factors combined to raise the issue up the policy agenda. First, Professor Knight chose to highlight this and other disparities on the info-graphic summary of the report (Figure 14.3). Advances in technology and graphic design, and the advent of social media, meant that infographic summaries were used for each MBRRACE-UK report and were disseminated widely. Second, the stark reality of the '5x' graphic led to immediate attention and a huge rise in advocacy from many support groups, both Black women's groups and more widely, who have continued to drive action.

Third, the coincidental timing of the Black Lives Matter protests, sparked by the death of George Floyd in the United States, brought this to the forefront of UK policymakers' attention. While a similar disparity had been noted and acted on in the United States, up to this point there had been an unvoiced assumption in the UK that disparity of this extent could not exist within the NHS, free to all at the point of access.

Challenges still to be tackled: structural and cultural biases

The spotlight on ethnic inequalities was shone even more brightly during the COVID pandemic, during the early months of which a rapid study from the UKOSS showed that more than half of pregnant women admitted to hospital with COVID-19 were from ethnic minority groups. Almost all women who died were from Black or Asian ethnic groups, and the Enquiry identified a number of areas where messaging about self-isolation and when to seek help could be strengthened, particularly for women with difficulties with English. The story

Key messages
from the report 2018

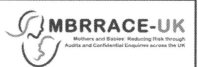

MBRRACE-UK
Mothers and Babies: Reducing Risk through
Audits and Confidential Enquiries across the UK

In 2014-16 **9.8** women per 100,000 died during pregnancy or up to six weeks after childbirth or the end of pregnancy.

Most women who died had multiple health problems or other vulnerabilities.

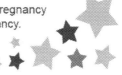

Balancing choices:

Always consider individual benefits and risks when making decisions about pregnancy

Things to think about:

Many medicines are safe during pregnancy

Continuing medication or preventing illness with vaccination may be the best way to keep both mother and baby healthy - ask a specialist

Black and Asian women have a higher risk of dying in pregnancy

White women		8/100,000
Asian women	2x	15/100,000
Black women	5x	40/100,000

Older women are at greater risk of dying

Aged 20-24		7/100,000
Aged 35-39	2x	14/100,000
Aged 40 or over	3x	22/100,000

Be body aware - some symptoms are normal in pregnancy but know the red flags and always seek specialist advice if symptoms persist

Overweight or obese women are at higher risk of blood clots including in early pregnancy

Figure 14.3 Infographic summary of the 2018 Report

of COVID-19, however, also illustrates some of the ongoing challenges for the Enquiry in addressing structural and cultural biases that impact care for pregnant women.

As is common practice, pregnant women were excluded from all initial trials of COVID vaccines, even those using established technologies which had been used to make other vaccines safely administered in pregnancy. Under emergency licensing arrangements no requirements were put in place with the companies concerned to undertake such trials. Existing mechanisms of ad hoc voluntary safety reporting of administration in pregnancy were initially relied upon to collect information on the outcomes of COVID vaccination. For several months after the start of the immunisation programme the fact of pregnancy at the time of vaccination was not recorded. Because of the lack of comprehensive data on vaccination safety in pregnancy, high levels of vaccine hesitancy remained among the pregnant population.

While pregnant women with COVID-19 were included in some treatment trials, the Enquiry found that many of the women who died had not received multidisciplinary care because teams were not co-located. The women were treated late or not at all with medical therapies shown to be effective in COVID-19. Often there was clear evidence that the treating doctors were concerned about fetal exposure, losing sight of the need for life-saving treatment for the woman herself. This echoes the patterns seen in breast cancer and epilepsy, with an overwhelming cultural focus on fetal risk without consideration of the benefits of treatment to women.

Structural biases restricting pregnant women's participation in vaccine trials led to lack of safety data and low levels of vaccine uptake. This, together with cultural biases denying them the best evidence-based treatments, led to continuing deaths of pregnant women in the third wave of infection in the UK in mid-2021. The fact that more women died during the third wave than either the first or second waves of infection, at a time when mortality rates were falling in all other population groups, emphasises the work still needed to ensure women's lives are saved.

How women's lives will continue to be saved

The 2020 Report illustrated the 'constellation of biases' (Figure 14.4) which continues to impact women's care before, during and after pregnancy (Figure 14.2). With more women entering pregnancy at older ages, and with more medical and mental health comorbidities, it is essential to ensure that they receive equitable care despite being pregnant, and the role of the Enquiry becomes ever more important. 'Treat a pregnant woman as you would

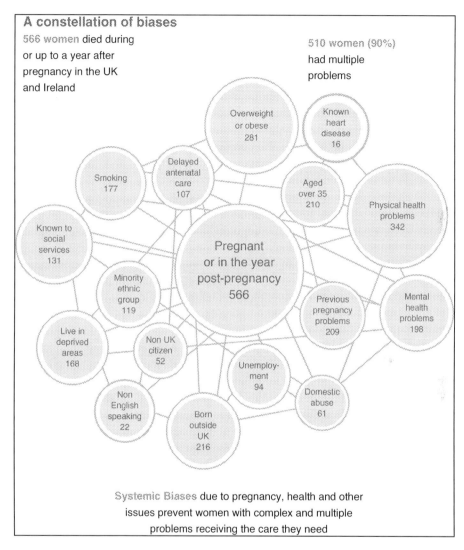

Figure 14.4 How biases interact

a non-pregnant person unless there is a clear reason not to' is perhaps the single most important message from recent Enquiries.

Consequent on the Enquiries' success in preventing maternal deaths due to obstetric causes is the need to ensure that their messages reach a much wider audience, including women and their clinicians, long before the woman becomes pregnant. It also includes doctors and nurses caring for pregnant women outside the maternity unit and policymakers and regulators in a wide variety of spheres. It is imperative to ensure that there are no barriers to communicating the findings. Investigation of the care of women who have had a 'near-miss' undoubtedly adds value and may, paradoxically, be the place to start to save women's lives in jurisdictions where maternal mortality enquiries are difficult. Nevertheless, as the examples in this chapter show, even after the dramatic successes of the CEMD in the twentieth century, its importance to saving lives remains in the twenty-first.

15 INTERNATIONAL MATERNAL HEALTH: GLOBAL ACTION

Avoidable maternal deaths during pregnancy or birth have always been a global problem. The World Health Organization (WHO) estimated that in the year 2000 more than half a million women died from pregnancy-related causes – roughly one death a minute. Most of those could have been prevented at little or no extra cost. The burden lies heaviest in the poorest countries of the world, and among the poorest of their poor. While some countries have made huge efforts to save their mothers, in general efforts over the past 30 years have been fragmented and by no means universal.

Previous chapters of this book have described a current UK picture that is still less than perfect, but the situation in low- and middle-income countries remains very much worse. This chapter shows how reviews are essential to making pregnancy safer and describes some of the methods the WHO recommends. In the next chapter doctors from different continents describe their experience of setting up Confidential Enquiries in their own countries – in South Africa, in the state of Kerala in India, which has achieved the lowest maternal death rate by far of any state in that populous country, and in the progressive and successful state of California in the USA. All these authors played leading roles within their national or statewide organisations, but here each of them is writing in a personal capacity.

Global action

In the 1990s the Safe Motherhood Movement and a number of advocacy groups such as the White Ribbon Alliance started to raise national and global awareness of the appalling figures surrounding maternal deaths, and the publicity eventually led to concerted international action (Figure 15.1).

In 1995 the United Nations (UN) set an ambitious, though ultimately unrealistic, Millennium Development Goal which was signed off by more than 160 countries (Figure 15.2). They all agreed to aim at reducing their maternal mortality ratio (MMR) by 75% by 2015, from its baseline in 1995.

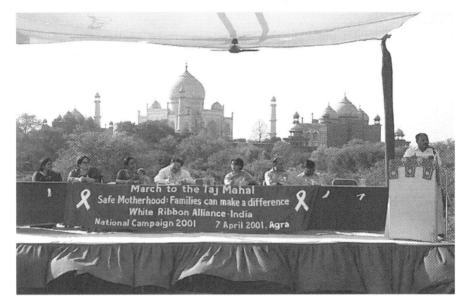

Figure 15.1 In 2001 women of the White Ribbon Alliance India marched from Delhi to Agra to raise awareness of maternal mortality. The Taj Mahal, built by a grieving Shah Jahan to honour Mumtaz Mahal, his beloved wife who died in childbirth, is the world's greatest monument to a mother's death.

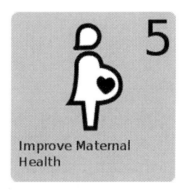

Figure 15.2 1995: Millennium Development Goal 5: to reduce maternal mortality by 75% by 2015

The MMR is defined as the number of mothers who die per 100,000 live births. Predictably the target proved far too challenging although the overall ratio did fall by around 43% globally and by more than that in a few African and Asian countries. But still the WHO estimated in 2017 that another 295,000 potentially avoidable maternal deaths occurred in that year – 810 a day.

The original target was superseded in 2015 by another equally ambitious – and probably equally unachievable – objective. Target 3.1 of the UN Sustainable Development Goals aimed to 'reduce the global MMR to less than 70 per 100 000 births, with no country having a maternal mortality rate of more than twice the global average' (Figure 15.3). In 2020 the average MMR for low-income countries was around 462 deaths per 100,000 live births, and the target to reduce this by nearly 80% was only 10 years away. By contrast, using the same international criteria, the MMR for the UK in 2016–18 was already only 4.1 maternal deaths per 100,000 live births.

More than 95% of the mothers who die are from two areas: Sub-Saharan Africa and southern Asia. The risk of a woman in a low-income country dying from a maternity-related cause is 130 times higher than for a woman from a high-income country. Despite the valiant efforts of underpaid, undervalued and under-resourced maternity staff in the worst-affected countries, these figures remain a global disgrace.

The mothers who suffer non-fatal complications

The gap in MMR between rich and poorer counties is already the largest public health discrepancy in the world, but it is compounded by the numbers of women who survive avoidable or treatable life-threatening conditions. The WHO estimates that, for every woman who dies, another 30 will face very

Figure 15.3 2015: Sustainable Development Goal 3.1: to reduce the global MMR to 70 deaths per 100,000 live births by 2030

severe problems, leaving many of them with long-lasting consequences such as vaginal fistula, incontinence, infertility and anaemia.

The real figures are probably far higher and take no account of the millions of women who suffer severe mental illness, some of whom will have died as a result. In most countries postnatal depression, suicide from puerperal psychosis and other mental health issues are not even acknowledged as pregnancy-related problems.

The babies who die

Babies are greatly affected by their mothers' health in pregnancy or during birth. Despite significant improvements over the past two decades, in 2019 more than 2.5 million babies were stillborn and around another 2.5 million died shortly after birth. Many more were left motherless and less able to thrive. Most of these babies' deaths were due in part to maternal conditions and, again, the vast majority died in Sub-Saharan Africa and southern Asia.

For a woman's existing children under the age of five, the risk of death is doubled if she dies in childbirth and is even worse for girls, who often remain the lowest of the low in the family hierarchy in terms of access to healthcare, education and adequate nutrition. If universal access to effective maternal and reproductive healthcare were available to all women, more than 14,000 babies' and 800 mothers' lives might be saved every day. This total of 5.5 million avoidable deaths each year far outweighs those from malaria, tuberculosis, human immunodeficiency virus (HIV) and other infectious diseases combined.

How to save lives

The main causes of maternal death in low- and middle-income countries are the same as those that used to predominate in the UK – bleeding, infection, high blood pressure, obstructed labour and unsafe abortion. Deaths from such 'direct' causes (entirely related to pregnancy) are now almost non-existent in the UK and generally can be prevented by simple, cheap and effective clinical interventions which have been available for many years.

Saving mothers' lives does not require high-tech facilities, expensive drugs or groundbreaking technology. What is needed is easier access to free or affordable essential maternal and newborn healthcare services which provide evidence-based, technologically appropriate and inexpensive interventions. Access to modern methods of contraception alone could prevent more than half of all maternal deaths. All of these actions are feasible today, even in the poorest countries of the world.

But concerted action is also needed to understand and address the wide range of underlying socially determined factors which lead to such inequalities in maternal health outcomes. This requires a multi-agency effort. At a national level, saving the lives of pregnant women does not depend on the easy rhetoric often spouted at national and international meetings by politicians with little or no action to back up their fine words. It depends on real political will and sustained efforts across the board.

In each country success relies on the priority given to mothers' and newborns' lives by those in positions of power and influence. It requires the upholding of the basic human right for all women to have universal access to reproductive and maternity health services. This right is still sadly lacking in some places. As the renowned father of the Safe Motherhood Movement, Professor Mahmoud Fathalla, presciently said at its launch in 1987: 'Mothers are not dying because of diseases we cannot treat. They are dying because societies have yet to make the decision that their lives are worth saving.'

'The only game in town'

Professor Fathalla has been described as 'unarguably the greatest Women's Health Rights champion of the last century'. A graduate of Cairo University, he gained his PhD in Edinburgh, became a professor of obstetrics and gynaecology in Assiut, Egypt and, in 1994, was elected president of the International Federation of Obstetrics and Gynaecology (Figure 15.4). He asked similar questions to those the UK Confidential Enquiries into Maternal Deaths (CEMDs) have also long sought to answer:

Why are our mothers dying?

What are the real, underlying reasons why they are dying?

What other factors apart from the quality or availability of healthcare or resources are contributing to their deaths or complication rates?

What barriers do women have to overcome as they journey along their pregnancy pathway? And what needs to be done to help?

He stressed the need for confidential reviews of all maternal deaths, like the UK CEMD, so remedial actions could be taken and lessons learned. Indeed the UK CEMD is referred to as the global gold standard to which other countries have long aspired. Prof. Fathalla underlined this in a speech in 2017 at the Royal College of Obstetricians and Gynaecologists:

As an old timer, I want to acknowledge the inspiring role of the College in the early days of the Safe Motherhood initiative. In those early days of the global awareness about the magnitude of this neglected tragedy, we did not have the rich information which we have today. But we were inspired by the work of the Royal College in setting up the system of 'Confidential Inquiry' and in reducing maternal death. In fact, for us then, it was the only game in town.

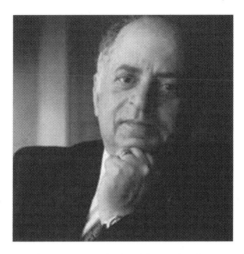

Figure 15.4 'I had the privilege to serve the health needs of women in parts of the world where people are poor and women are the poorest of the poor. In my professional career there is no more tragic event than a maternal death. For those of us practising in developing countries, maternal mortality is not words and is not numbers. It is women who have names. It is about human faces seen in the throes of agony, distress and despair. Faces that live forever in our memory and continue to haunt our dreams. These are young women in the prime of their lives who die at a time of joy and expectation, leaving behind children and families in real need of their care.'
Professor Mahmoud Fathalla

Beyond the Numbers

As awareness grew of the benefits of going deeper into the real reasons why mothers died – and acting on the lessons learned – in 2004 the WHO published a practical toolkit, *Beyond the Numbers: Reviewing Maternal Deaths and Complications to Make Pregnancy Safer* (BTN) (Figure 15.5). Although now superseded by a later programme which rightly includes perinatal deaths, the *Maternal and Perinatal Death Surveillance and Response* (MPDSR) programme, BTN's main principles remain the foundation for all of this work. *Beyond the Numbers* described four approaches to learning lessons from reviewing the stories of mothers who died or suffered severe complications, and these can be used at any level, nationally or locally, in any country, rich or poor. While it drew on experience from other countries, it was mostly written and edited by the director of the UK CEMD. The four approaches range from the local to the national:

- Facility-based deaths reviews
- Community-based death reviews ('verbal autopsy')
- Near-miss, or severe obstetric morbidity enquiries
- National (or regional) confidential enquiries into maternal deaths

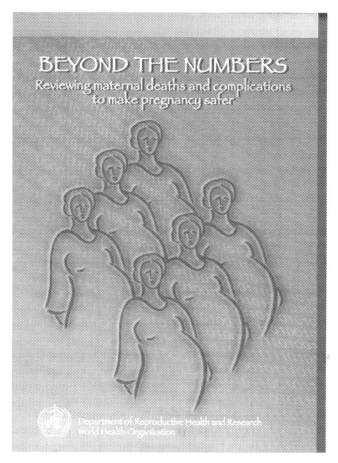

Figure 15.5 Avoiding maternal deaths is possible, even in resource-poor countries, but it requires the right kind of information.

Knowing the level of maternal mortality is not enough; we need to understand the underlying factors that led to these deaths.

Each maternal death or case of life-threatening complication has a story to tell and can provide indications on practical ways of addressing the problems.

A commitment to act on the findings of these reviews is a prerequisite for success. From the Preface of *Beyond the Numbers*.

Each approach is discussed in what follows, but all four need to be practical, acceptable and effective. The full support of health professionals, administrators and policymakers is essential, and it must be crystal clear from the outset that action must be taken on the results. Otherwise the considerable efforts to introduce the reviews will be wasted and staff support and advocacy in future will be lost. This philosophy of acting on results is re-emphasised in the title of the later MPDSR, where the use of the term 'response' emphasises this requirement.

The early reaction

The maternal health world seemed to have been waiting for BTN. Following its launch in Kenya in 2004, the roll-out was quick. The WHO and sister organisations such as the United Nations International Children's Emergency Fund (UNICEF) and the United Nations Fund for Population Activities (UNFPA) held regional and in-country workshops at which each country developed its own plan for the implementation of its chosen approach. Representatives of professional organisations and ministries of health from more than 100 countries attended these events, and many of these representatives then formed national maternal health committees as a first step towards developing and implementing their chosen programmes. Some achieved significant improvements.

Initially countries wanted to implement nationwide confidential enquiries along the lines of the CEMD, but most were ill prepared to do so. Developing a CEMD from scratch involves winning the hearts and minds of sceptical – if not alarmed – health professionals, and this takes time and effort. It was soon recognised that it was better to 'start small' and then build the system up. The approach eventually chosen by virtually everyone was to develop a system to learn lessons from the mothers who died in health facilities, as these deaths were far easier to identify and the data were easier to collect. The aim was to expand these local systems and, once they were working well, to cover wider areas or entire countries, although that does not seem to have happened to date.

Local reviews

Facility-based reviews take place weekly or monthly depending on the numbers of cases, and the staff consider the lessons to be learnt from problems encountered in their own hospital. They are really an extension of 'grand rounds', the regular maternal and neonatal audit meetings which have been held for many years in hospitals whose lead professionals take seriously the issues of safety, quality of care and learning lessons.

Community-based reviews are necessary for the smaller number of women who die outside hospital. These reviews are far more challenging and require specifically trained local staff. It is hard to identify women who are unknown to health services, let alone get a comprehensive and medically correct history of their illness. In some places such women are seen by their family as having died from the effects of spells or evil spirits.

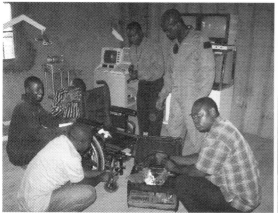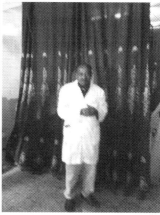

Figures 15.6 and 15.7 The repair shop and the saris

Hospital reviews may be carried out by an anonymised paper-based system but usually mothers' deaths and complications are discussed at staff meetings. There can be of great benefit in learning together and identifying local solutions for local problems but the meetings need careful management to enable the staff to speak freely and without fear of blame. In the past it was all too easy to scapegoat junior staff, especially those who were not present, or the long-suffering midwives who were rarely invited to attend the meetings.

Once that easy option is discarded, the avoidable factors that emerge are generally not due to the actions of one person, but to a lack of teamwork, clinical guidelines, resources or staff training. Identifying these factors, however, is only the beginning of the process.

How to do it - and how not to do it
In one trailblazing African hospital an initially successful review programme eventually failed because no action was ever taken on the results. The leading health professionals claimed to be committed to making changes to clinical care but they did not follow through. Likewise the hospital administrators failed to change rotas, refurbish clinics or allocate the required resources. The staff, originally enthusiastic, became so disillusioned that they stopped participating in future enquiries and actively discouraged others from doing so. Further avoidable deaths followed.

These problems, however, can be managed with care and attention. Facility-based reviews are still the most widely used system in the world today and can promote significant achievements. One example, among many, is a hospital in Ethiopia where the staff also went out into the surrounding communities to talk to relatives about the factors leading to the mothers' deaths. They identified issues such as a lack of blood supplies, an ambulance which had been commandeered by the police (an all-too-common finding elsewhere) and reluctance among mothers to come to hospital because of lack of privacy and a perception that the staff were hostile and abusive.

These findings resulted in a dedicated ambulance and an altruistic blood bank provided by other inpatients. Rotas were improved so staff were less tired and developed a more respectful attitude to women. The unit's director provided saris to act as curtains for privacy in labour and the whole facility was cleaned and made more welcoming. Rather than wait for donors to replace or repair broken equipment (which can take years), a partnership was developed with the local technical college. This provided students with training and job opportunities – as well as income generation from other hospitals whose equipment had also failed. Clinical guidelines and protocols followed, and other departments were so impressed with the reduction in mothers' deaths that they introduced similar reviews.

Near-miss reviews

As mentioned, women who survive severe life-threatening complications outnumber those who die by around 30 to 1. For those with less catastrophic complications the ratio is more than 100 to 1. In countries where the numbers of maternal deaths are too small to provide a solid basis for identifying trends, BTN implementation has therefore tended to focus on 'near-miss' reviews. The larger data sets allow more robust analyses and provide stronger evidence to support recommendations.

Other advantages are that mothers can add their own observations and staff can congratulate themselves on 'great saves', as near-misses are called in the South African Enquiries. The larger numbers also allow more frequent and responsive reporting. In the UK the MBRRACE system provides an annual update on key topics (see Chapter 14).

National Enquiries in smaller countries

In smaller countries with relatively low death rates, such as those in the Balkans and some ex-Soviet states, another problem is confidentiality. Numbers of maternal deaths are often low enough to make it possible to identify each mother and her carers. This is of particular concern in countries where healthcare workers have traditionally faced punishment or prison if a woman died, even if their care had been the best possible in the circumstances. Naturally they are reluctant to tell the truth, even anonymously, unless there are legal assurances. The necessary institutional shift takes time, however, and the cultural shift takes even longer before the staff feel able to report the true facts of the case.

One option in these circumstances is to greatly expand the numbers by instituting a near-miss review. Another is for adjacent countries with similar demographics and healthcare systems to join together, widening their pool of cases. This is why Scotland, Northern Ireland and eventually the Republic of Ireland joined the UK CEMD. The Scandinavian enquiries run on broadly the same lines and the Baltic States may possibly do the same.

Confidential Enquiries before *Beyond the Numbers*
Even before confidential enquiries were widely promoted by the WHO, a few enlightened obstetricians had established such systems in their own countries, some as far back as the 1970s. Most of them had spent time working in the UK and had seen the strengths of the CEMD approach. These enquiries were more common in higher-income countries such as Australia, New Zealand, Canada, France and Italy, and in Scandinavia, where the willingness and capacity to undertake such in-depth reviews were available, but there were notable exceptions such as Egypt, Kerala, Sri Lanka and South Africa. Each of these countries had a well-established professional association, some form of national health service to provide equitable care for all mothers and a system not dominated by private obstetric practice.

Most of the lower-income countries and states which developed sustainable confidential enquiries not only had supportive staff and professional associations, but also had socialist or ex-communist governments when their CEMDs started. Kerala and Sri Lanka, for example – resource-poor places with impressively low maternal death rates – both have traditions of seeking to treat girls equally with boys and free access to every level of education and healthcare services.

Confidential Enquiries after *Beyond the Numbers*
In the years since the publication of BTN in 2004, only a few confidential enquiries have been properly and sustainably introduced. It has become clear from the detailed debates about which approach to adopt – and from bitter experience – that a country's prospects for introducing even simple facility-based reviews depend on many interconnecting issues, not all of them healthcare based, and that the challenges are much greater for confidential enquiries.

The first requirement is sound data. A national review depends on a fully functioning system for the collection of comprehensive, reliable and up-to-date statistics, and a robust mechanism for identifying all maternal deaths, wherever they occur. This is often impossible, but lessons may still be learnt from smaller reviews of maternal deaths or near-misses, through the use of specially designed protocols. These local facility-based death or near-miss reviews are currently the main legacy of BTN in most parts of the world.

The second requirement is the full support and engagement of all relevant health professionals, administrators and local stakeholders. They all need education and training before an enquiry can be implemented. Without this, enquiry programmes, even with good-quality data systems, are not sustainable,

At a national level, governmental backing is required. This means fully supporting the process, ensuring staff support and engagement, providing adequate resources and making a real commitment to act on the findings and recommendations.

Finally, but most importantly, all staff must feel able to participate without risking punishment or adverse effects. They need to know their anonymity and confidences will be respected and that their contribution will be used to improve maternal health outcomes. This means removing legal or other obstacles to the maintenance of confidentiality. In many places, however, this lesson has still to be learned.

Lessons learned: blame

In some countries it is mandatory to report maternal deaths to the police so the alleged perpetrators can be immediately arrested. Fingers may be pointed at innocent staff by upset relatives, and senior staff may blame each other, their juniors and the midwives. There is an ingrained assumption that a mother's death is always caused by the negligence of individuals rather than by a lack of clinical guidelines, training or resources. None of this is conducive to frank discussions about the real circumstances of the mother's death or to learning lessons for improving care. Failures are usually systemic and the solutions are service-wide.

A recent paper on why maternal death reviews have failed in India states that, despite pockets of good practice, a pervasive culture of blame and denial persists within a corrupt, uncaring system. 'Studies have routinely indicated that medical staff repeatedly blamed the auxiliary nurse-midwives for errors . . . and referred women with life threatening conditions to other facilities in order to avoid being blamed for maternal deaths.'

Also, in some places, there is still a regrettable tendency to blame the mothers for their own deaths. In a developed Middle Eastern country the expert medical assessors of a series of local facility reviews decided that one-third of the mothers had brought their 'misfortune' on themselves. This assertion was not challenged by their peers or the Ministry of Health. The project was scaled up, with no apparent understanding of why the system was failing, and continues to harm mothers.

Fear and confidentiality

Confidentiality is the first line of defence against blame and dishonest reporting. Many promising enquiries have faltered when assurances about the maintenance of confidentiality failed. The fear of being named and blamed is very real and results in demoralisation and obfuscation. This makes it impossible to determine the real chain of events and the lessons that need to be learnt and acted upon. A UK report into improving safety in the NHS, when discussing professional reluctance to engage in audits and reviews, memorably concluded: 'Fear is toxic to both safety and improvement.'

'To err is human': developing a safety culture

The benefits of developing a culture which encourages learning to improve quality and safety – rather than punishment and blame – was underlined by the publication of *A Promise to Learn, a Commitment to Act*, issued by the Department of Health in England in 2013. 'Because human error is normal and, by definition, unintended, well-intentioned people who make errors or [work] in systems that have failed around them need to be supported, not punished, so they will report their mistakes and the system defects they observe, so that all can learn from them.' This ethos has always underpinned the UK Confidential Enquiries, but sadly it is still poorly understood in many countries today.

Professionalism

Why do some obstetricians fail to support or participate in the reviews described here? Would 'arrogance' be too strong a word? In some countries – especially, it seems, those where the majority of doctors choose to work in private practice – confidential enquiries have never really taken off. Or lip service may be paid to their principles by supporting their introduction in the public-sector hospitals, leaving private facilities immune from review. This pattern is seen everywhere – in low- and high-income countries and those in between. A lack of reflective learning and an 'I know best and don't need guidelines' attitude remain sadly pervasive.

What works

We know maternal death and near-miss reviews, and confidential enquiries, work. The success of CEMDs from different parts of the world and under various circumstances is described by their own directors in the next chapter. But we know too that unless planned carefully and supported widely – by staff, administrators, policymakers, government, women, media and the public – they can fail, and badly. But despite the warning lessons described in this chapter, experience has shown they really do save lives.

Over time the most successful reviews have been characterised by three interdependent, supportive factors, each of which contributes to a positive and enabling environment. These are:

- 'A maternity conscience' where there is individual altruistic responsibility, professionalism, support and ownership by all healthcare workers, whether they are involved in being honest when completing the forms or assessing the cases, or through promoting and implementing the subsequent recommendations.
- A 'facilitative institutional ethos' where the managers of each health facility proactively promote and encourage learning as a crucial part of improving services and quality of care.
- A 'supportive and facilitative political and policy environment'.

When all three levels – political, institutional and individual – work together, women's lives can be saved.

16 INTERNATIONAL ACTION: PERSONAL VIEWS

Section 1: Implementing Confidential Enquiries into Maternal Deaths in South Africa

ROBERT PATTINSON

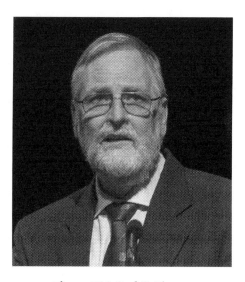

Figure 16.1 Prof. Pattinson

South Africa in the mid-1990s was an optimistic country brimming with new ideas and hope for the future. We were initially blessed with leaders of foresight. The minister of health, Dr Dlamini-Zuma, was a medical doctor with a scientific background, and together with the director general of health, Dr Ayanda Ntsaluba, and the director of maternal and child health, Dr Eddie Mhlanga (both O&G specialists), he responded positively to a request by clinicians in South Africa for the establishment of Confidential Enquiries into Maternal Deaths (CEMDs) based on the UK model. In 1997 Prof. James Drife was invited out to give guidance on getting started.

The background

The idea of a confidential enquiry was not new in South Africa. Prof. Elsa Boes collected information on maternal deaths from throughout the country in the late 1970s and early 1980s. She entitled her thesis 'Too Little, Too Late'. In 1981 Prof. Alan Rothberg established an annual meeting of obstetricians, neonatologists, paediatricians, midwives, doctors working in rural areas, community health specialists and members from the Department of Health, all working mostly in the public sector. This group was one of the key elements in establishing the CEMD and dispersing the information.

One of the tasks the group members set themselves was to set up an investigation into maternal deaths in the country. Members from each province were tasked with approaching their bosses to try to initiate the investigation. The reply I received from the Transvaal director general of health in 1991 was negative and I was prohibited from visiting or communicating with any other hospitals. Without political support a CEMD cannot be initiated.

The beginning

In 1997 Minister Dlamini-Zuma appointed a committee with Prof. Jack Moodley as chairperson and a system of forms adapted from the UK CEMD was created and distributed to all hospitals. A decentralised system of collecting and analysing the cases was devised. In each of the nine provinces was a provincial CEMD committee comprised of a member of the national committee and assessors from every district. No assessor could assess deaths from his or her own district. Doctors and nurses with skills in obstetrics for at least five years were appointed in every province. Every death was assessed by a doctor and midwife.

The minister and her team facilitated the process further by two actions: making a maternal death a notifiable condition and reaching an agreement with the Department of Justice that the information obtained by the CEMD would be kept confidential. The woman's file is owned by the woman and her family, and they can at any time request the file from the hospital and take it to any lawyer if they want to litigate.

The Maternal Death Notification Form (MDNF) and the assessor's form were part of the property of the Department of Health and they could not be, and never were, asked for by the families. Recently, however, the Protection of Personal Information (POPI) Act, effective from July 2020, has made this agreement redundant. However, the national committee's standard operating procedures demand that the documents are shredded every three years to ensure confidentiality and the only documents left were the Saving Mothers reports. For this reason the comprehensive Saving Mothers reports were top heavy with detailed tables as the report served as the only reference document.

The first Report

In January 1998, with all the stars aligned, the process started and the first report was produced for just that year, again under the supervision of Prof. James Drife, and presented to the National Department of Health (NDoH) and at the Priorities Conference in 1999. The findings were then also presented in every province and district, often by the assessors. This ensured the information spread to all corners of South Africa. The report was also published and sent to all stakeholders, so there was an effective method of dissemination.

Developments followed fairly rapidly thereafter with a national electronic database being developed by Dr Johan Coetzee with multiple security features. The provinces started entering the data and a streamlined system of reporting and assessing developed, allowing for a rapid production of reports within six months after the end of the year in question. National assessors' workshops were held to train assessors and ensure a constant standard of assessment. Further a quality controller was appointed in each province who would randomly assess approximately one in five cases and give feedback to the assessors. Recommendations were refined in such a way that their implementation and impact could be measured.

The HIV/AIDS epidemic

However, the halcyon days did not continue. In the 2000s the country was being overwhelmed by the HIV/AIDS epidemic. Unfortunately, in South Africa, the president (Thabo Mbeki) and minister of health (Manto Tshabalala-Msimang) were AIDS deniers. They were supported by some officials in the NDoH. Thus when presenting the 2005–7 findings to the minister of health we were chased out of the minister's office for mentioning HIV/AIDS and NDoH members tried to alter the report such that HIV/AIDS was not mentioned.

The publication of the 2005–7 report was delayed a few years, but the comprehensive report still contained all the details. There was one positive aspect to this event: the minister complained that 'we never bring her any good news, only bad news'. This is true – a CEMD, by definition, only discusses deaths, never 'great saves'. This led to more attention being put on developing a maternal near-miss system so one would not only discuss deaths, but could also say how many lives the system saved!

In 2008 a new minister of health (Barbara Hogan) was appointed, who was replaced shortly thereafter by Dr Aaron Motsoaledi, and both were supported by the deputy director general and head of programmes, Dr Yogan Pillay. The CEMD now enjoyed more attention and the recommendations were incorporated into the national strategic plan. Maternal deaths peaked in 2009, with an in-facility maternal mortality rate (iMMR) of 300/100,000. In 2019 it was 97/100,000.

The effects of the CEMD

The CEMD had many positive spin-offs. The new minister of health liberalised the use of antiretroviral drugs for treating HIV. The rapid reporting led to detection of nivirapine (one of the antiretroviral drugs used for treatment of pregnant women with HIV) as toxic. Once identified, and with the efficient system of feedback, the protocols were changed and a sudden reduction in maternal deaths due to adverse drug reactions was recorded.

A second example of the value of the CEMD was the identification of bleeding at or after caesarean delivery (CD) as a major cause of maternal death and increasing problem. At one stage more than a third of all maternal deaths due to obstetric haemorrhage were due to bleeding at or after CD. This problem was addressed by training and developing and introducing the Safe CD programme. There has been a significant tail-off in this as a cause of death in the last triennial report.

Other interventions initiated due to findings and recommendations by the CEMD (e.g. the Essential Steps in Managing Obstetric Emergencies pro-gramme), together with emergency obstetric simulation training exercises, were introduced and made compulsory for all interns prior to registration. The standard antenatal care pack, which had been based on the World Health Organization (WHO)–focussed African National Congress system with reduced visits, was changed when it became apparent there had been an increase in maternal deaths due to hypertension.

Improving the process

The CEMD has produced seven triennial reports plus annual reports. A useful exercise was conducted in the mid-2010s when the NDoH organised a review of the process by Prof. Heather Scott to identify weaknesses and make recom-mendations to improve the process. This led to the annual reports being more substantial. The last development has been the integration of the perinatal review committee's reports to produce the *Saving Mothers and Babies* report with integrated recommendations.

The Maternal and Perinatal Death Surveillance and Response (MPDSR) system promoted by the WHO has always been a part of the CEMD system. Each case is discussed locally (within the district) and any action that needs to be immediately taken can be taken by the authorities. The MDNF and copy of the file is still sent to assessors and the cases confidentially assessed. The strength of this is that rarer occurrences can be detected and acted on. In my view the CEMD should be in the hands of a professional body such as the Colleges of Medicine in South Africa or the South African Medical Research Council (SAMRC). This will preclude the NDoH from dictating to the committee and refusing to publish the reports as has happened in the past.

Summary

Success due to health administrators and clinicians with vision (all levels), a vast network to distribute information rapidly, a decentralised system which leads to local buy-in, emphasis on confidentiality and an electronic database which allows for rapid reporting: all of these factors led to the documentation of a two-thirds reduction in the iMMR from 2009 to 2019.

Section 2:   The Kerala Experience

VAKKARAM PAILY

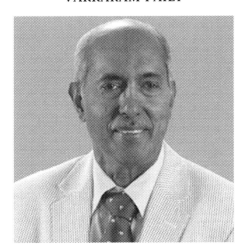

Figure 16.2 Dr Paily

Kerala has a low maternal mortality rate (MMR) compared to other states in India. Credit for this belongs to several groups or agencies. The foundation was laid decades ago by rulers of the state who promoted female literacy. Subsequent rulers continued to improve the standard of living by introducing land reforms, establishing schools, laying roads, building hospitals and providing health infrastructure.

When the Kerala Federation of Obstetrics and Gynaecology (KFOG) was founded in 2002 we collaborated with the government of Kerala in planning and executing projects aimed at reducing the MMR. This section outlines the steps we took in the hope this summary will be useful for other countries, states and communities and their obstetricians.

Maternal death audit

The first requirement for reducing maternal mortality in any setting is to find out the details of maternal deaths. How many mothers have died? What were the circumstances of their deaths? What were the medical and other underlying reasons? The answers can be known only by proper audit, and the WHO described the various methods in its monograph *Beyond the Numbers*:

1.   Confidential enquiry into (review of) all maternal deaths
2.   Near-miss reviews of those mothers who suffered life-threatening complications

3. Facility-based audit: deaths occurring in a health facility
4. Verbal autopsy; deaths in the community

Which type suits a particular setting depends on various factors. For confidential enquiries, proper documentation (complete case records) is essential and the same is more or less true for near-miss and facility-based audits. Verbal autopsy, however, is usually done by interviewing family and healthcare workers to ascertain the sequence of events, and this can be done in the absence of case records. It is suitable for maternal deaths occurring in the community or in health facilities with few staff members and poor infrastructure.

Confidential Review of Maternal Deaths (CRMD) in Kerala

Confidential Enquiry into Maternal Deaths (CEMD) has been going on in the UK for nearly 70 years. It is acclaimed as the gold standard of maternal death audit and its findings have revolutionised obstetric care not only in the UK, but globally. Its special feature is its anonymisation of records. Also no punishment or reprimand is given even if a lapse in the management is identified. The aim is to learn lessons and rectify omissions and commissions so deaths can be avoided in similar circumstances in future. Following the UK experience, many countries started confidential enquiries with minor modifications but sticking to the principle of confidentiality and a non-punitive nature.

The KFOG decided to implement confidential review of maternal deaths in the same pattern as the UK. This process is suitable because Kerala has nearly 98% institutional deliveries, a privilege many other states in India do not have, and confidential review is possible only if a case record is available. However, we brought in some changes and, instead of 'enquiry', we called it 'review' (CRMD instead of CEMD). We were able to convince the Department of Health of Kerala of the usefulness of the process and the government offered full support.

In the UK the CEMD has now evolved into Mothers and Babies: Reducing Risk through Audits and Confidential Enquiries (MBRRACE) (see Chapter 14), which audits not only maternal deaths, but near misses and other obstetric events, including stillbirths and infant deaths. In Kerala we too have progressed from CRMD by modifying the process and decentralisation (see later in this chapter). We have moved on to confidential near-miss audits in our medical colleges, but the CRMD continues.

Initial steps

In 2002 the KFOG had decided to audit all maternal deaths in the state, but in 2003 a training workshop organised in Delhi by the WHO gave the final push to start. The WHO also supported a workshop in Thiruvananthapuram, the capital city of Kerala, to disseminate the idea among health department officials and senior obstetricians of the state. Professor Gwyneth Lewis, the director of the UK Enquiry, attended to share her experience and to explain how to overcome any challenges. After this the government of Kerala authorised the KFOG to conduct the review and told all hospitals, private and governmental, to hand over anonymised case records of maternal deaths to the KFOG.

Organisation of the audit team

The Maternal-Fetal Medicine (MFM) Committee of the KFOG was given the responsibility of conducting the audit and its chairperson (VP Paily) was made the state coordinator of the CRMD. A large group of senior and middle-level obstetricians were trained to conduct the audit and designated as assessors. An executive committee was formed, consisting of 14 senior assessors drawn from the different segments of healthcare – medical colleges, other government hospitals and private hospitals. All the assessors, senior as well as middle level, were instructed to keep strict confidentiality.

Data collection

Four forms were developed to report the details of the maternal death:

Form A contains the identifying details of the deceased. It is subsequently destroyed.

Form B carries no identifying information about the patient, the hospital or the doctor. It is marked by a code number assigned by the state coordinator.

Form C is completed by the team from the district medical office who will be doing the facility-based audit in every institutional maternal death.

Form D is filled by the treating obstetrician and sent directly to the state coordinator. It has information which the obstetrician wants to share in strict confidence, such as lapses in management or suggestions for management that might have changed the outcome. This form allows the obstetrician to ask for confidential feedback from the coordinator after the audit is over. There will be no chance of adverse consequences for the honest obstetrician who realises his or her lapses and wants to learn from the feedback.

In addition to these forms a photocopy of the anonymised case records is sent to the state coordinator.

Maintaining anonymity

The state coordinator generates a code number and separates Form A (with the names) from the other forms. The code number is marked in all other forms and case records and Form A is filed separately in a very secure place. Photocopies of the case records are taken after masking all identifying features including the address of the deceased. They are put in a large cloth-lined envelope and marked with the code number.

The process of auditing

All case files, with Form B, are sent out for audit by the assessors. Usually every case is sent to one member of the executive committee and one of the other assessors. As far as possible care is taken to see that cases are sent to assessors located far away from the place where the death occurred. The assessors are reminded each time to maintain confidentiality. There is a separate form for them to enter their findings. The assessed records are sent back to the state coordinator. We often need expert comments from non-obstetrician specialists and we have a pool of volunteers among the cardiologists, anaesthesiologists, neurologists, nephrologists, gastroenterologists, physicians and so forth.

Quarterly review

Once every three months the assessors meet on a Sunday to review the cases audited in the previous months. The coordinator makes a summary of the cases which is circulated to all participants. Those who reviewed the cases present their findings and the entire team joins the discussion. The non-obstetrician assessors also are requested to join the meeting. After discussion a cause of death is assigned to each case and a comment is made as to whether it was avoidable and whether there was undue delay at any stage of care.

The meeting is scheduled by turn in the north, south and centre of the state. The local obstetricians and postgraduate students are invited to attend as observers. The audit team members are rotated, with new members recruited to replace those who stand down after long periods. No honoraria or travel expenses are paid to the assessors. The KFOG meets the expenses and no financial support is sought from the government.

Dissemination of information

The KFOG publishes the findings of the audit as a book. The first edition was entitled *Why Mothers Die – Kerala 2004–05* and the second edition covered the period 2006–9. Copies are given free to all KFOG members and are available for free download from the KFOG website (http:kfogkerala.com). The third edition, covering the period 2010–19, was published in January 2022.

Compilation and publication of the results takes a long time. To ensure that lessons are passed on to practitioners without delay, learning points from each quarterly meeting are printed in the KFOG journal and circulated among the members across the state.

An overall perspective of the medical reasons for maternal death is compiled and disseminated to practising obstetricians and authorities. Haemorrhage is the leading killer of mothers and hypertension is the second commonest cause. Other contributors are heart disease, pulmonary embolism, amniotic fluid embolism and sepsis.

Follow-up actions

Audit is meaningless unless one acts on the findings, especially when these relate to public health. As well as identifying the causes of maternal deaths we developed strategies to address the underlying issues, particularly regarding major remediable causes such as bleeding, high blood pressure and infection. The fact that in Kerala nearly all mothers give birth in a health facility allowed us to target the obstetricians, nurses and paramedical staff.

However, we identified an unbelievably large number of locations where mothers gave birth, both in the governmental and in the private sector. Many did not have 24-hour facilities or staff to care for women during or after labour, especially if complications occurred. Blood banks were very few and situated only in the large cities, and the unavailability of blood and blood products was a big problem, especially in the outlying areas. Blood component therapy was scarce. Maternity transport was a big hurdle as there was no organised ambulance service.

Many changes in practice were required. For example, aseptic techniques to prevent infection were not practised in many centres and had to be promoted widely. Caesarean delivery rates were rising in the government and private sectors and this had to be addressed. The knowledge base of the obstetricians and nurses had to expand, attitudinal changes were required and facilities had to improve.

How to bring about changes in practice

The KFOG alone could not bring about these changes. The government of Kerala had to be approached, and its Department of Health was very proactive. The Department of Health agreed to our suggestions to conduct training workshops for doctors and nurses. The KFOG drew up the curriculum and provided the trainers. Practical issues had to be overcome in arranging training sessions for peripheral health workers. Although private hospitals accounted for 70–80% of deliveries there was initial reluctance to train private-sector staff using government funds. Nevertheless training sessions were conducted in all districts for government and private hospital staff, though sometimes KFOG had to solicit funding for these from pharmaceutical companies.

Involvement and education of pregnant women and their families are essential to reduce maternal deaths and disabilities. Kerala has the inherent advantage of high female literacy and we decided to promote antenatal classes in all delivery centres. We thought this would help pregnant women to understand any complications that might arise, enable them to identify when they needed to seek help and reduce delays accessing skilled care.

Emergency obstetric care and life support

The audit revealed that many deaths were due to the lack of emergency obstetric care at the right time. A recurring feature was that staff working in more peripheral locations lacked either the facilities to provide appropriate emergency care or the knowledge to identify when the mother needed to be transferred. By the time she is brought to a higher-level centre, valuable time has been lost. These issues were not limited to the small peripheral centres, however. Even in bigger centres a lack of timely help in emergencies was obvious.

Practical training was needed to address this problem and we conceived the Emergency Obstetric Care and Life Support (EMOCALS) project. On completion of training, the trainees received a certificate valid for five years. We soon realised that obstetricians and nurse midwives have different training needs, and we divided the training into EMOCALS-D (doctors) and EMOCALS-N (nurses). The government gave financial support for this scheme.

Quality standards in obstetric care

In 2012–13 the health secretary of the state of Kerala invited NICE International (part of the UK National Institute for Heath and Care Excellence) to get involved. They were impressed with what we had already done and, based on the findings of the CRMD, they helped us to develop the Quality Standards in Obstetric Care guidelines, focussing on the main causes of maternal death. Simple but enforceable standards were developed to address the problem of deaths due to postpartum haemorrhage and hypertension.

These included active management of the third stage of labour, blood transfusion, observation in intensive-care or high-dependency units and an ultrasound scan at 32 weeks for every woman who had had a previous caesarean section. We insisted on blood pressure checks at every antenatal visit and frequent urine testing, and gave detailed guidelines on treatment of pregnancy-induced hypertension. These messages were taken to all obstetricians through training programmes.

The Quality Standards project was piloted in eight hospitals and the results were gratifying, with a marked change in the referral pattern of patients from the periphery. The project was then expanded to other districts. Similarly, NICE helped us to draft quality standards for the management of amniotic fluid embolism, sepsis and heart disease. The collaboration was reported in an international journal but the scheme faltered due to changes in the government department and a shortage of funding.[*]

Near-miss audit

With the total number of deaths in the state being fewer than 180 per year, many hospitals would have very few cases – or none at all – from which to learn lessons. We therefore decided to audit 'near-miss' cases, where women survived life-threatening complications. In 2014 the government of India published operational guidelines on maternal near-miss audit. We followed these but, unlike our counterparts in other countries, we decided also to follow the principles of confidential audit in near-miss cases. A pilot project was started with the five major government medical colleges in Kerala and the process is still going on.

Other initiatives

We also established obstetric rapid response teams to prevent complications progressing to a critical stage. Obstetricians and nurses were trained in emergency obstetric care and at least one trained person has to be in the labour

[*] VP Paily, K Ambujam, V Rajasekharan Nair, B Thomas, 'Confidential review of maternal deaths in Kerala: a country case study'. *BJOG* 2014;121Suppl 4:61–6. https://doi.org/10.1111/1471-0528.13000.

room around the clock. These individuals are identified by badges and are given special drugs and equipment. Basic life support skills and airway management also are taught. Workshops to train labour room faculty (doctors and nurses) were conducted in all districts with support from the government of Kerala.

We thought it important to devolve the centralised audit process to the district level, with a local convenor and chair, in a project called the Maternal Death and Near Miss Surveillance and Response (MDNMSR). The obstetricians of the district started to meet on a monthly basis to discuss serious obstetric problems, including deaths and near-miss cases, without revealing women's identities. These events gave peripheral obstetricians the opportunity to identify local solutions and also turned out to be a forum for academic exchange. Technical innovations included new instruments for use in catastrophic obstetric haemorrhage, which helped to change the outcome of post-partum haemorrhage.

A state target and national recognition

By 2018 we felt that declaring a target would help our efforts to gain momentum. The Kerala government agreed and made a public declaration of its commitment to achieve MMRs of 30 (per 100,000 births) by 2020 and 20 by 2030. It sounded ambitious but achievable and the KFOG joined with the state government to work towards the goal.

The success of the CRMD in Kerala was noted at the national level. Two representatives were invited to participate in discussions when the government of India developed its Maternal Death Surveillance and Response (MDSR) guidelines, which now include CRMD as one of the strategies.

An unexpected twist: suicide deaths on the rise

We were on course to achieve the target until 2019–20, when there were 19 maternal deaths from suicide. This had been a matter of concern since the CRMD started but in the early years suicide was counted as a 'fortuitous' cause and excluded from the calculation of MMR. In 2012, however, the WHO recommended including it as a direct cause. In other developed countries like the UK suicide is now recognised as a leading cause of maternal death and work has shown that deaths linked to acute post-partum psychosis can be prevented. The government of Kerala has started a project called Amma Manass and the KFOG has encouraged studies of the social and psychological problems faced by pregnant and postnatal women. The KFOG has encouraged its members to start antenatal classes in all delivery centres to help young pregnant women cope with the stresses of pregnancy.

Conclusions[†]

In 2019 there were 131 maternal deaths in Kerala, according to data from the director of health services, and 475,184 births, giving an MMR of roughly 28. It therefore appears that we have achieved the target MMR of 30. How? There have been several factors but we believe the focussed attempt of the KFOG to bring down the MMR played a major role. More than anything, we instilled a sense of commitment in all the obstetricians – including those in the private sector – to work with the government to achieve this goal. Much more, however, remains to be done. Haemorrhage, hypertension and sepsis are still the leading causes of maternal deaths in the state. Continued vigilance and concerted efforts are needed to sustain the achievements.

Importantly, CRMD Kerala and all the activities aimed at reducing maternal deaths were possible only with the full support of the government of Kerala and an army of obstetricians and non-obstetrician colleagues across the state. Society at large should be grateful to all these committed health workers, including nurses, paramedics, public health staff and Asha workers and administrators, for their selfless services.

[†] This is an edited version of 'Measures to reduce maternal mortality: the Kerala experience' by VP Paily, K Ambujam, B Thomas, PK Sekharan and V Rajasekharan Nair, published in *Update obstetrics and gynaecology 2021*, edited by Pratibha Devabhaktuni and S Rani Reddy, chapter 5, pages 86-92. Published by Paras Medical Books. ISBN:978-8195271535.

Section 3:   Maternal Mortality Reviews to Action: California Successes and Challenges

ELLIOTT MAIN, MD

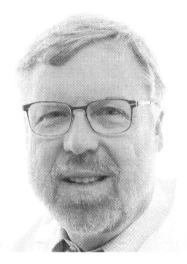

Figure 16.3 Dr Main

The California maternal mortality experience can be told as a personal story, as an institutional history or as part of a national narrative. All have been heavily influenced by the UK Confidential Enquiries. As a medical student interested in obstetrics in the 1980s I was awed by the wonder of a normal birth juxtaposed by the horror of a maternal death. I read about each and every triennial CEMD report in *The Lancet* and was heavily influenced by Fred Frigoletto's case series of maternal catastrophes in the *New England Journal of Medicine*. During a career in maternal-fetal medicine caring for the sickest of mothers, I gradually shifted focus from clinical medicine to quality improvement, leading system improvements first at the level of a large maternity hospital (5,000 annual births), then at the level of a large healthcare system (45,000 annual births), and finally for the state of California (450,000–500,000 annual births). At each level we sought to take lessons from individual cases to highlight and drive evidence-based system changes that improved care for all future mothers. The need for system-level improvements was one of the key lessons learned from the CEMD.

Background

California has the largest population (40 million) and by far the largest number of births of any state in the United States, accounting for one of every eight US births. American healthcare is highly decentralised so that each state makes its own laws and regulations, collects its own vital statistics and has its own insurance plans. The exceptions that are handled at the federal level are Medicare (health insurance for retirees) and regulations for medications. Given the relative rarity of maternal deaths in high-resource countries (10–20/100,000 live births), having so many births in a single administrative jurisdiction provided an important opportunity both to better understand maternal deaths in the United States and to develop and test large-scale quality improvement (QI) initiatives. But, at the start, California historically did not even have a maternal mortality review committee.

Review committees

Maternal mortality review committees as an important tool to reduce US maternal mortality were initiated in the city of Philadelphia in the 1930s. Subsequently they were initiated in many large states and cities. With the rapid fall in maternal deaths throughout the 1950s and 1960s, many committees closed in the late 1970s. In the early 2000s US maternal deaths began to rise. In 2006 the California Department of Public Health noted that California maternal deaths appeared to also be rising and established the California Pregnancy-Associated Mortality Review Committee (CA-PAMR). The state was very interested in translating the findings into improvement actions and asked that I lead the committee and establish the California Maternal Quality Care Collaborative (CMQCC) to undertake large-scale maternal QI. This began our 15-year journey to change maternity outcomes at scale.

We decided initially to focus on pregnancy-related mortalities and our committee was composed accordingly with nurses, midwives, social workers and physicians representing obstetrics, maternal-fetal medicine, emergency medicine, anaesthesia, cardiology and other specialties as needed. More recently we have included community members and persons with lived experience. Subcommittees with different specialties have examined maternal deaths from suicide and substance use.

Since we were already thinking about the next steps, we specifically asked in each case review 'What were the improvement opportunities demonstrated in this case?', making it straightforward to collect and analyse themes. It became evident early that two common causes of maternal mortality – obstetric haemorrhage and hypertensive disorders – had high frequencies (>90%) of provider improvement opportunities and therefore, also high rates of 'chance to alter the outcome'.[1, 2, 3, 4] We quickly realised that clear preventability was a difficult judgement given the limitations of data available for review (typically medical records and not interviews with staff or family). Nonetheless, these two categories of maternal mortality stood out as demanding immediate action and led to the development of the most important step in our California story – turning the review results into direct action.

Improvement initiatives

Soon after the formation of the CMQCC, we began testing approaches for large-scale QI initiatives. The very first project was not related to maternal mortality but to the reduction of early elective deliveries to reduce neonatal morbidity and mortality from scheduled births at 36, 37 and 38 weeks of gestation. This was an incredible success, with an 80–85% reduction within two years. Four key strategies were piloted that we have used in all QI initiatives since:

(1) Create a multidisciplinary QI toolkit for use by hospital staff to provide an evidence-based practical approach to addressing change.
(2) Establish a broad-based set of partner organisations to push together for improvement.
(3) Produce and promote a national performance measure that is reported by every facility.
(4) Create incentives for hospitals and providers to engage and want to improve. The incentives can be altruistic ('need to address high mortality rates) or financial (gain or loss) or both.

Toolkits and collaboratives

Our first CMQCC QI toolkits, *Improving Health Care Response to Obstetric Hemorrhage* (now in its second edition),[5] and *Improving Health Care Response to Hypertensive Disorders of Pregnancy* (also in its second edition),[6] were immediately followed by a series of QI collaboratives modelled after the IHI Breakthrough Series with multidisciplinary teams at each hospital who met for a 'kick-off' in-person meeting followed by group monthly phone check-in sessions to review barriers and strategies as well as brief reviews of content from the toolkits. The collaboratives grew from including 20 hospitals to 56 hospitals to a maximum of 130 hospitals (California has 235 hospitals with maternity services and >98% of births occur in hospital). To best serve hospitals

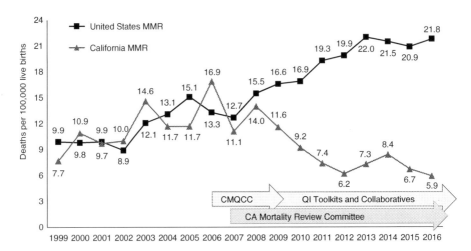

Figure 16.4 California, 1999–2016. The CMQCC was established in 2006 and maternal mortality reviews started in 2007 with QI toolkits and collaboratives following in 2009.
CA-PMSS Surveillance Report: Pregnancy-Related Deaths in California, 2008–2016.
Sacramento: California Department of Public Health, Maternal, Child and Adolescent Division, 2021.
www.cdph.ca.gov/Programs/CFH/DMCAH/surveillance/Pages/CA-PMSS.aspx

in the large collaboratives we divided the hospitals into groups of 8–10 with paired nurse and obstetrician QI mentor/coaches.[7] This approach was very well received and has become our standard.

Over the first five years, California's maternal mortality rate fell from 14–17 (equal to the United States as a whole) to 6–7 per 100,000 births, similar to other high-resource countries. These data are illustrated in Figure 16.4.

Other maternal QI toolkits that have been released have covered cardiovascular diseases, sepsis, mother-baby substance exposure and supporting vaginal birth/reducing primary caesareans (all are open source and available at www.cmqcc.org/resources-tool-kits/toolkits).

The Maternal Data Center

In 2012 we introduced the fifth key strategy – the CMQCC Maternal Data Center – that combines the clinical data from birth certificates (provided from the Department of Public Health within 30 days after delivery) with hospital discharge data files and with limited hospital-sourced clinical data. The Maternal Data Center has multiple goals: (1) provide benchmarking for more than 90 measures against like hospitals; (2) provide rapidly available metrics to support

QI initiatives; (3) provide low-burden data to use for reporting to multiple different external organisations. This has proven extraordinarily popular and now serves three states in the western United States with more than 300 hospitals.

The latest QI initiative that was heavily dependent on the Maternal Data Center was a statewide effort to lower the caesarean rate for first-birth mothers. This was important, as the high US rate for primary and repeat caesareans is associated with significant maternal morbidity. High caesarean rates have been notably difficult to reduce but with our five strategies we were able to reduce the rate from 26% (the same as the United States) to four percentage points lower, meeting the national 2030 target.[8]

Severe maternal morbidity

As the number of maternal deaths is so low even in such a large state as California, we have focussed our QI efforts on major complications or Severe Maternal Morbidity (SMM) as defined by the Centers for Disease Control. For example, in our haemorrhage collaborative work among hospitals, our focus is on the reduction of SMM among women with haemorrhage. Similarly for the hypertension collaboratives we used SMM among women with hypertensive disorders. This has allowed hospitals to identify measurable improvement within a shorter period and allows the MDC to use these metrics for surveillance after the collaborative is completed.[9]

Federal action

The accomplishments in California have spurred national efforts to use similar approaches in other states. Federal funding has been provided to develop comparable perinatal quality collaboratives and they are now off the ground in a total of 44 of the 50 states. Federal support has also gone the American College of Obstetricians and Gynecologists to support multidisciplinary teams to develop national safety bundles on the same topics for which the CMQCC produced QI toolkits. These bundles are short checklists of actions every hospital should adopt and are supported by many other national organisations. The CMQCC staff and physicians have led or contributed to the development of each of these national bundles.[10]

Continuing collaboration

Today, as we continue to evolve and improve our processes, we carefully review each new report of the successor organisation to the CEMD, MBRRACE-UK

(Mothers and Babies: Reducing Risk through Audits and Confidential Enquiries). There are significant challenges as we move beyond addressing the classic direct causes of maternal mortality. As maternal deaths are now more often in the late post-partum period or very early in gestation, more importance is placed on outpatient care and the role of non-obstetric providers. The gap between Black and Native American women and other racial groups has been difficult to close. The effect of social determinants requires collaboration with other government programmes and a more holistic view of health. If there is one overarching lesson from all the years of CEMD it is that reduction of maternal mortality and severe morbidity requires constant surveillance and effort by many partners.

FIGURE PERMISSIONS

The authors are very grateful to the following organisations and individuals for granting permission to publish the Figures listed below.

Cambridge University Press

Figures 3.2 and 4.2 are from Names and Eponyms in Obstetrics and Gynaecology, 3rd ed. (2019), by Professor Thomas Baskett (who took the photograph at Figure 4.2).

Confidential Enquiries into Maternal Deaths

Figure 5.5 is republished from Why Mothers Die 2000–2002, the Sixth Report of the Confidential Enquiries into Maternal Deaths in the United Kingdom (page 110).
Figure 6.2 is reproduced from the CEMD Report for 1964–66 (page 21).
Figure 8.2 is reproduced from the CEMD Report for 1952–54 (page 23).
Figure 8.7 is republished from Why Mothers Die 2000–2002 p110, the Sixth Report of the Confidential Enquiries into Maternal Deaths in the United Kingdom (page 104).
Figure 9.5 is reproduced from Why Mothers Die 1997–1999: the Confidential Enquiries into Maternal Deaths in the United Kingdom. London, RCOG Press 2001 (page 51).
Figure 9.6 is reproduced from Saving Mothers' Lives: Reviewing maternal deaths to make motherhood safer: 2006–2008. BJOG 2011;118 Suppl 1:1–206 (page 58).
Figure 10.1 was redrawn from data in: Saving Mothers' Lives: Reviewing maternal deaths to make motherhood safer: 2006–2008. BJOG 2011;118 Suppl 1:1–206. With grateful thanks to Professor Jason Gardosi at the Perinatal Institute for Maternal and Child Health.
Figure 10.2 is reproduced from Why Mothers Die 2000–2002: the Sixth Report of Confidential Enquiries into Maternal Deaths in the United Kingdom. London: RCOG Press, 2004 (page 139).
Figure 13.3 is the front cover of the CEMD Report for 1994–96.

Elsevier

Figure 9.1 is reproduced from: Greer IA, Thomson AJ. Management of venous thromboembolism in pregnancy. *Best Practice & Research Clinical Obstetrics and Gynaecology* 2001;15(4):583–603.

Getty Images

Figure 8.1 is a photograph by George W. Hales, published by arrangement with Fox Photos/Hulton Archive/Getty Images.
Figure 8.3 is published by arrangement with McCabe/Express/Hulton Archive/Getty Images.

Glasgow Royal Infirmary

Figure 8.6 is reproduced by permission of the Medical Illustration Services, Glasgow Royal Infirmary.

Guardian/Eyevine

Figure 8.4, copyright Martin Argles/GNM, is reproduced by arrangement with Eyevine.

Institute of Psychiatry

Figure 3.6 is reproduced by permission of the Institute of Psychiatry, London.

Lancet / Elsevier

Figure 3.1 is reproduced, with permission, from Sir George Godber's obituary in The Lancet of 7th March 2009 (volume 373, page 804).

MBRRACE

Figures 13.4 and 13.5 are from the MBRRACE Report, *Saving Lives, Improving Mothers' Care 2016–2018.*
Figure 14.2 is reproduced from the 2017 CEMD Report.
Figure 14.3 is reproduced from the 2018 MBRRACE Report.
Figure 14.4 is reproduced from the 2020 MBRRACE Report

National Portrait Gallery

Figure 2.5 is from the National Portrait Gallery (public domain)

Oxford University Press

Figure 5.4 is reproduced by permission from *"The Tragedy of Childbed Fever"* by the late Dr Irvine Loudon, published in 2000.

Professor Tom Clutton-Brock

Figure 11.3 was kindly provided by Professor TH Clutton-Brock.

Royal College of Midwives

Figure 1.3 is reproduced by permission of the Royal College of Midwives.

Royal College of Obstetricians and Gynaecologists

Figure 3.5 is reproduced from: RCOGM/P0035, Sir John Peel (1904–2005), KCVO, President of the Royal College of Obstetricians and Gynaecologists (1966–1969), with the permission of the Royal College of Obstetricians and Gynaecologists

Figure 6.1 is reproduced from: RCOGM/P0031, Dame Hilda Lloyd (1891–1982), DBE, President of the Royal College of Obstetricians and Gynaecologists (1949–1952), with the permission of the Royal College of Obstetricians and Gynaecologists

Figure 9.3: Front Cover and Table 5: Risk Assessment Profile for Thromboembolism in Caesarean Section are reproduced from 'Report of the RCOG Working Party on Prophylaxis against Thromboembolism in Gynaecology and Obstetrics' (RCOG,1995), with the permission of the Royal College of Obstetricians and Gynaecologists

University of Aberdeen

Figure 8.5 is reproduced by permission of the Special Collections Department, University of Aberdeen.

University of Chicago

Figure 7.1 is reproduced by permission of the University of Chicago.

Wellcome Collection

Figures 1.1, 1.4, 1.5, 2.1, 2.3, 11.1 and 13.1 are in the public domain at wellcomecollection.org/images.

Figures 5.2, 5.6, and 5.8 are reproduced with special acknowledgement to the Wellcome Collection.

World Health Organization

Figures 15.2, 15.3 and 15.5 are reproduced by permission of the World Health Organization.

Other figures

Figures 2.6, 3.3, 3.4, 8.8, 9.2, 12.2, 12.3, 12.4, 13.2, 13.6, 13.7, 13.8, 14.1, 15.1, 15.4, 15.6, 15.7, 16.1, 16.2, 16.3 and 16.4 were each provided by the author of the relevant chapter. Other Figures are in the public domain and/or out of copyright.

FURTHER READING

1 Historical Background

Campbell JM. Maternity homes. Lancet 1921;198(5017):163–4.

Dunn PM. The Chamberlen family (1560–1728) and obstetric forceps. Archives of Disease in Childhood: Fetal and Neonatal Edition 1998;81:F232–F235.

Halliday J, Halliday S. Zepherina Veitch (1836–94): childbed fever and the registration of midwives. Journal of Medical Biography 2007;15:241–5.

Loudon I. Death in childbirth: an international study of maternal care and maternal mortality 1800–1950. Oxford: Clarendon, 1992.

Shaw WF. Sir Francis Champneys. BJOG 1948;55(3):312–17.

Shaw WF. The birth of a college. BJOG 1950;57(6):877–89.

Smellie W. A treatise on the theory and practice of midwifery. London: Bailliere Tindall, 1752. Reprinted by Hansebooks, 2018.

Wilson A. The making of man-midwifery: childbirth in England 1660–1770. Cambridge, MA: Harvard University Press, 1995.

2 The First Steps

Editorial. The maternal mortality of childbirth and the teaching of midwifery. Lancet 1919;193(4993):802–3.

Editorial. Maternal mortality. Lancet 1934;224(5803):1111–12.

Hogarth M. Dame Janet Mary Campbell (1877–1854). Oxford Dictionary of National Biography. Oxford: Oxford University Press, 2006. https://doi.org/10.1093/ref:odnb/32267

Holland E. Maternal mortality. Lancet 1935;225(5926):973–6.

Loudon I. The transformation of maternal mortality. BMJ 1992;305(6868):1557–60.

MacLennan H. The pioneer spirit. BJOG 1965;72(4):530–4.

Maternal mortality and morbidity: final report of [the] Departmental Committee. BMJ 1932;2(3736):327–9.

Obituary: Andrew Topping. Lancet 1955;266(6888):511–13.

Topping A. Maternal mortality and public opinion. Public Health 1936;9:342–9.

3   How the Confidential Enquiries Evolved

Anderson M. Changing childbirth: commentary I. BJOG 1993;100(12):1071–2.

Chalmers I, Enkin M, Kierse MJNC. Effective Care in Pregnancy and Childbirth. Oxford: Oxford University Press, 1989.

Department of Health. Changing childbirth. Part I: report of the Expert Maternity Group. London: Her Majesty's Stationery Office, 1993.

Dunlop W. Changing childbirth: commentary II. BJOG 1993;100(12):1072–4.

Editorial. Preventing maternal deaths. Lancet 1957;270(6991):375.

Editorial. The Cranbrook Report. Lancet 1959;273(7069):397–8.

Godber G. AJ Wrigley (obituary). British Medical Journal 1984;288:415.

Godber G. The origin and inception of the Confidential Enquiry into Maternal Deaths. BJOG 1994;101(11):946–7.

Lewis G, ed. Saving mothers' lives: reviewing maternal deaths to make motherhood safer: 2006–2008. The Eighth Report of the Confidential Enquiries into Maternal Deaths in the United Kingdom. BJOG 2011;118 Suppl. 1;1–203. [As of February 2022, this report had been cited 1,857 times in the general literature and in 457 academic papers.]

Lewis G, Drife J. Why Mothers Die 1997–99: the Confidential Enquiries into Maternal Deaths in the United Kingdom. London: RCOG Press, 2001.

Lewis G, Drife J, Botting B et al. Why Mothers Die: report on Confidential Enquiries into Maternal Deaths in the United Kingdom 1994–1996. London: TSO, 1998.

Paintin D. Commentary: effective care in pregnancy and childbirth. British Journal of Obstetrics and Gynaecology 1990;97(11):967–73.

Weindling AM. The Confidential Enquiry into Maternal and Child Health (CEMACH): a review of the history of Confidential Enquiries. Archives of Disease in Childhood 2003;88:1034–7.

4   The Missing Chapter?

Barry CN. Home versus hospital confinement. Journal of the Royal College of General Practitioners 1980;30(211):102–7.

Editorial. Current practice in obstetrics. British Medical Journal 1964;1(5383): 580.

Jeffcoate TNA. Prolonged labour. Lancet 1961;278(7193):61–7.

MacLennan HR. The management of labour in contracted pelvis. British Medical Journal 1954;2(4892):837–40.

Miller D. Common obstetrical injuries and their sequelae. British Medical Journal 1936;2(3939):4–6.

O'Driscoll K, Jackson RJA, Gallagher JT. Prevention of prolonged labour. British Medical Journal 1969;2(5655):477–80.

Sheehan HL. Shock in obstetrics. Lancet 1948;251(6488):1–7.

Wood LAC. Obstetric retrospect. Journal of the Royal College of General Practitioners 1981;31(223):80–90.

5 How the Change Began

Buddeberg BS, Aveling W. Puerperal sepsis in the 21st century: progress, new challenges and the situation worldwide. Postgraduate Medical Journal 2015;91 (1080):572–8.

Colebrook L. Prevention of puerperal sepsis: a call to action. British Medical Journal 1936;1:1257–9. [Colebrook had long campaigned for better aseptic practice in childbirth. This heartfelt paper appeared in the BMJ two weeks after his historic *Lancet* report on prontosil.]

Colebrook L, Kenny M. Treatment of human puerperal infections, and of experimental infections in mice, with prontosil. Lancet 1936;227(5884):1279–81.

Duka T. Childbed fever, its causes and prevention: a life's history. Lancet 1886;128 (3283 and 3284): 206–8 and 246–8. [These articles about Ignaz Semmelweis were written by Theodor Duka, who restored his reputation.]

Loudon I. The tragedy of childbed fever. Oxford: Oxford University Press, 2001. [This is the definitive history of puerperal sepsis.]

Lowis GW, Minagar A. Alexander Gordon of Aberdeen and the contagiousness of puerperal fever. Journal of Medical Biography 2002;10:150–4.

Noble WC. Coli: great healer of men. The biography of Dr Leonard Colebrook FRS. London: Heinemann, 1974.

Obstetrical Society of London. Discussion on puerperal fever. Lancet 1875;105 (2698):685–92.

6 Haemorrhage Then and Now

Black MD. Blood transfusion in obstetrics. British Medical Journal 1937;1(3082):903–6. (and correspondence in British Medical Journal 1937;1(3084):1043–4).

Hendry J, Baird D. Treatment of placenta praevia. Transactions of Edinburgh Obstetrical Society 1937;57:25–44.

Liang DYS. The emergency obstetric service, Bellshill Maternity Hospital 1933–1961. BJOG 1963;70(1):83–93.

Lloyd HN et al. Discussion on [the] emergency obstetrical service (the flying squad): its use and abuse. Proceedings of the Royal Society of Medicine 1949;42:1–10.

Mavrides E, Allard S, Chandraharan E, et al. on behalf of the Royal College of Obstetricians and Gynaecologists. Prevention and management of postpartum haemorrhage. (Green-Top Guideline No. 52.) BJOG 2016;124:e106–e149.

Pavord S, Rayment R, Madan B et al. on behalf of the Royal College of Obstetricians and Gynaecologists. Management of inherited bleeding disorders in pregnancy. (Green-Top Guideline No. 71: Joint with UKHCDO.) BJOG 2017;124:e193–e263.

Thomson AJ, Ramsay JE, on behalf of the Royal College of Obstetricians and Gynaecologists. Antepartum haemorrhage (Green-Top Guideline No. 63). London: Royal College of Obstetricians and Gynaecologists, 2011.

WHO recommendations for prevention and treatment of postpartum haemorrhage. www.who.int/reproductivehealth/publications/maternal_perinatal_health/9789241548502/en

7 Hypertension

Eclampsia Trial Collaborative Group. Which anticonvulsant for women with eclampsia? Evidence from the Collaborative Eclampsia Trial. Lancet 1995;345:1455–63.

Magpie Trial Collaborative Group. Do women with pre-eclampsia, and their babies, benefit from magnesium sulphate? The Magpie Trial: a randomised placebo-controlled trial. Lancet 2002;359:1877–90.

National Institute for Health and Care Excellence. Hypertension in pregnancy: diagnosis and management. NICE Guideline 133, 2019. www.nice.org.uk/guidance/ng133

WHO recommendations for prevention and treatment of pre-eclampsia and eclampsia. www.who.int/reproductivehealth/publications/maternal_perinatal_health/9789241548335/en

8 The Story of Abortion

Abortion and maternal deaths. British Medical Journal 1976;2(6027):70.

Anonymous. The statistics of 100 cases of abortion. Lancet 1902;159:1125–6.

Anonymous. Should abortion be legalised? Lancet 1932;219:627.

Anonymous. A charge of illegal abortion: Rex v. Bourne. Lancet 1938;232:220–6.

Baird D. A fifth freedom? British Medical Journal 1965;2(5471):1411–18.

Davis A. 2,665 cases of abortion: a clinical survey. British Medical Journal 1950;2(4671): 123–30.

Diggory PLC. Some experiences of therapeutic abortion. Lancet 1969;293:873–5.

Drife J. Historical perspective on induced abortion through the ages and its links with maternal mortality. Best Practice & Research Clinical Obstetrics and Gynaecology 2010;24:431–41.

General Medical Council. Deputation on the Midwives Bill. British Medical Journal 1895;1(1796):1244–7.

Malleson J. Criminal abortion: a suggestion for lessening its incidence. Lancet 1939;233:366–7.

On the frequency of criminal abortion. Provincial Medical Journal 1843;2:471–2.

Rowlands S (ed.). Abortion care. Cambridge: Cambridge University Press, 2014.

Thomson AT. Lectures on medical jurisprudence now in the course of delivery at the University of London: Lecture XVII: on abortion. Lancet 1837;27:625–30.

9 Challenging Tradition

Asher R. Talking sense. London: Pitman, 1972.

Atlee HB. Evidence in favour of a more active puerperium: a study of 500 cases. Canadian Medical Association Journal 1935;33(2):144–50.

Bryant EC. Early ambulation in the practice of obstetrics. Canadian Medical Association Journal 1947;57(3):257–9.

Drife J. Deep venous thrombosis and pulmonary embolism in obese women. Best Practice & Research Clinical Obstetrics & Gynaecology 2015;29(3):365–76.

Editorial. Early discharge of maternity patients. British Medical Journal 1964;2 (5401):70–1.

Hampton JR. The end of clinical freedom. British Medical Journal 1983;287 (6401):1237–8.

Royal College of Obstetricians and Gynaecologists. Reducing the risk of venous thromboembolism during pregnancy and the puerperium. Third edition. (Green-Top Guideline No. 37a). London: Royal College of Obstetricians and Gynaecologists, 2015.

Salzman KD. The nature and some hazards of obstetrics in general practice. British Medical Journal 1955;2(4930):15–19.

Thomas J, Paranjothy S, RCOG Clinical Effectiveness Support Unit. National Sentinel Caesarean Section Audit Report. London: RCOG Press, 2001.

Thornton P, Douglas J. Coagulation in pregnancy. Best Practice & Research Clinical Obstetrics and Gynaecology 2010;24(3):339–52.

10 Pregnancy and Illness

Carapetis JR. Rheumatic heart disease in developing countries. New England Journal of Medicine 2007;357(5):439–41.

Drife JO. Breast cancer, pregnancy, and the pill. British Medical Journal 1981;283:778–9.

Head CEG, Thorne SA. Congenital heart disease in pregnancy. Postgraduate Medical Journal 2005;81:292–8.

Nelson-Piercy C. Handbook of obstetric medicine. Sixth edition. London: Routledge, Taylor & Francis, 2021.

Powrie RO, Greene MF, Camann W, eds. De Swiet's medical disorders in obstetric practice. Fifth edition. Chichester: Wiley-Blackwell, 2010.

Schaufelberger M. Cardiomyopathy in pregnancy. Heart 2019;105:1543–51.

Soma-Pillay P, Nelson-Piercy C, Toppanen H, Mebazaa A. Physiological changes in pregnancy. Cardiovascular Journal of Africa 2016;27(2):89–94.

Yarris JP, Hunter AJ. Roy Hertz MD (1909–2002): the cure of choriocarcinoma and its impact on the development of chemotherapy for cancer. Gynecologic Oncology 2003;89:193–8.

Yentis SM, Steet PJ, Plaat F. Eisenmenger's syndrome in pregnancy: maternal and fetal mortality in the 1990s. British Journal of Obstetrics and Gynaecology 1998;105(8):921–2.

11 Maternal Death due to Anaesthesia

Sykes WS. Essays on the first hundred years of anaesthesia. Volume 2. 1982. Edinburgh: E&S Livingstone.

Grieff JMC, Tordoff SG, Griffiths R et al. Acid aspiration prophylaxis in 202 obstetric anaesthetic units in the UK. Int J Obstet Anesth. 1994;3:137–42.

Interim report of Departmental Committee on Maternal Mortality & Morbidity. London: His Majesty's Stationery Office, 1930.

Thomas J, Paranjothy S. Royal College of Obstetricians and Gynaecologists Clinical Effectiveness Support Unit: The National Sentinel Caesarean Section Audit Report. London: RCOG Press; 2001.

12 Psychiatric Illness

Cantwell R. Perinatal mental health service development across the UK: many achievements, growing challenges. Irish Journal of Psychological Medicine. (2022): 1–4. https://doi.org/10.1017/ipm.2022.1

Howard LM, Molyneaux E, Dennis C-L, Rachat T, Stein A, Milgrom J. Non-psychotic mental disorders in the perinatal period. Lancet 2014;384:1775–88.

Jones I, Chandra PS, Dazzan P, Howard LM. Bipolar disorder, affective psychosis, and schizophrenia in pregnancy and the post-partum period. Lancet 2014;384:1789–99.

Khalifeh H, Hunt, IM, Appleby L, Howard LM. Suicide in perinatal and non-perinatal women in contact with psychiatric services: 15 year findings from a UK national inquiry. Lancet Psychiatry 2016;3:233–42.

Oates M. The development of an integrated community service for severe postnatal mental illness. In Motherhood and Mental Illness 2: causes and consequences, ed. S Kumar and IF Brockington, pp. 133–58. London: Wright, 1988.

Prettyman RJ and Friedman T. Care of women with puerperal psychiatric disorders in England and Wales. British Medical Journal 1991;302:1345–6.

13   The Mothers Who Died

Department of Health. Inequalities in Health: report of an independent enquiry chaired by Sir Donald Acheson. London: Her Majesty's Stationery Office, 1998.

Department of Health and Social Security. Inequalities in Health: report of a research working group chaired by Sir Douglas Black. London: Department of Health and Social Security, 1980.

Godber G. The Confidential Enquiry into Maternal Deaths: A limited study of clinical results. In: A Question of Quality? Roads to assurance in medical care. Nuffield Provincial Hospitals Trust, ed. G McLachan, pp. 23–34. Oxford: Oxford University Press, 1976.

Gray A M. Inequalities in Health. The Black Report: a summary and comment. https://pubmed.ncbi.nlm.nih.gov/7118327

Lewis G, ed. Saving Mothers' Lives: the seventh report of the Confidential Enquires into Maternal Deaths in the UK. CEMACH. December 2007. www.cmace.org.uk

Lewis G, ed. Saving Mothers' Lives: the eighth report of the UK Confidential Enquiries into Maternal Deaths. Centre for Maternal and Child Health Enquiries. March 2011. Published as BJOG 2011;118Suppl1: 1–203. https://doi.org/10.1111/j.1471-0528.2010.02847.x

Marmot M. Health equity in England: the Marmot review ten years on. BMJ 2020;368:m693.

Marmot M, Allen J, Boyce T, Goldblatt P, Morrison J. Health equity in England: the Marmot review 10 years on. London: Institute of Health Equity, 2020. www.instituteofhealthequity.org/the-marmot-review-10-years-on

Oliver A. Reflections on the development of health inequalities policy in the United Kingdom. Working Papers 11/2008. LSE Health. London: School of Economics and Political Science, 2008.

Oxley WH, Phillips MH, Young J. Maternal mortality in Rochdale. British Medical Journal 1935;1(3867):304–7.

Socialist Health Association. The Black Report. 1980. www.sochealth.co.uk/national-health-service/public-health-and-wellbeing/poverty-and-inequality/the-black-report-1980

14   The Legacy in the UK

https://healthtalk.org/conditions-threaten-womens-lives-childbirth-pregnancy/ overview. This is a website with women describing their near-miss experiences.

Hinton L, Locock L, Knight M. Experiences of the quality of care of women with near-miss maternal morbidities in the UK. BJOG. 2014 Sep;121 Suppl 4 (Suppl4): 20–3. https://doi.org/10.1111/1471-0528.12800. PMID: 25236629; PMCID: PMC4312976.

Knight M, Acosta C, Brocklehurst P et al. Beyond maternal death: improving the quality of maternal care through national studies of 'near-miss' maternal morbidity. Southampton: NIHR Journals Library, 2016. PMID: 27386616.

Knight M, Bunch K, Vousden N et al. A national cohort study and confidential enquiry to investigate ethnic disparities in maternal mortality. EClinicalMedicine. 2021 Dec. 13;43:101237. https://doi.org/10.1016/j.eclinm.2021.101237. PMID: 34977514; PMCID: PMC8683666.

Knight M, Lindquist A. The UK Obstetric Surveillance System: impact on patient safety. Best Pract Res Clin Obstet Gynaecol. 2013 Aug;27(4):621–30. https://doi .org/10.1016/j.bpobgyn.2013.03.002. Epub 2013 Mar 30. PMID: 23548471.

www.thelancet.com/series/maternal-health-2016

Marshall O, Blaylock R, Murphy C, Sanders J. Risk messages relating to fertility and pregnancy: a media content analysis. Wellcome Open Res. 2021 May 14;6:114. https://doi.org/10.12688/wellcomeopenres.16744.1. PMID: 34286102; PMCID: PMC8276184.

15   International Maternal Health

Borchert M, Bacci A, Baltag V, Hodorogea S, Drife J. Improving maternal and perinatal health care in the Central Asian Republics. International Journal of Gynecology and Obstetrics 2010;110:97–100.

Fathalla M. Human rights aspects of safe motherhood. Best Practice and Clinical Research in Clinical Obstetrics and Gynaecology 2006;20(3):409–19.

Fathalla M. Reproductive rights and reproductive wrongs. Current Women's Health Reports 2001;1(3):169–70.

Lewis G. Reviewing maternal deaths to make pregnancy safer. Best Practice & Research Clinical Obstetrics and Gynaecology 2008;22(3):447–63.

Lewis G. Saving mothers' lives: the continuing benefits for maternal health from the United Kingdom (UK) Confidential Enquires into Maternal Deaths. Seminars in Perinatology 2012;36(1):19–26.

Lewis G. The cultural environment behind successful maternal death and morbidity reviews. BJOG 2014;121 Special issue 4 (International Reviews: Quality of Care):24–31.

Rosenfield A, Maine D. Maternal mortality, a neglected tragedy: where is the M in MCH? Lancet 1985;326(8446):83–5.

Say L, Chou D, Gemill A et al. Global causes of maternal deaths: a WHO systematic analysis. Lancet Global Health 2014;2:e323–e233.

Thaddeus S, Maine D. Too far to walk: maternal mortality in context. Social Science and Medicine 1994;38(8):1091–110.

World Health Organization. Trends in Maternal Mortality 2000 to 2017: estimates by WHO, UNICEF, UNFPA, World Bank Group and the United Nations Population Division. Geneva: World Health Organization, 2019.

World Health Organization, Lewis G. Beyond the Numbers: reviewing maternal deaths and complications to make pregnancy safer. Geneva: World Health Organization, 2004.

16   International Action

Professor Pattinson

For those interested in more details of the South African experience with CEMDs, the articles by Moodley and colleagues (2014) and Moodley and colleagues (2018) give more details. In an attempt to make the Saving Mothers reports more accessible, a number of the chapters from the seventh *Saving Mothers Report 2017–2019* related to conditions were published in the Obstetrics and Gynaecology Forum (https://journals.co.za/toc/medog/30/4).

There also some other spin-offs from a CEMD which are often not recognised, but very important. The system set-up allows for rapid recognition of complications which are rare but in a large enquiry become apparent, for example the article by Fawcus and colleagues (2016) highlighted the problem of deaths due to bleeding at or after caesarean delivery, which led to an immediate response. The system also can be used to rapidly report on new diseases such as COVID-19. Here the CEMD was able to produce quarterly reports to the ministerial committee working on COVID-19 and highlight for the committee the higher mortality of COVID-19 in pregnancy, putting pregnant women in the high-risk category and stressing their need for vaccination.

Finally, a CEMD is an integral part of the audit cycle. Poor-quality emergency care was identified early as a problem in maternal deaths by the CEMD in South Africa. Thus permission was obtained from Professor Nyncke van den Broek and the Royal College of Obstetricians and Gynaecologists to adapt their 'Life Saving

Skills' course to South African circumstances. The adapted course, 'Essential Steps in Managing Obstetric Emergencies', was tested in South Africa. Twelve of the worst-performing districts were identified using the CEMD. In partnership with the Liverpool School Tropical Medicine and their volunteers, the adapted course was scaled up in these 12 districts such that at least 80% of all healthcare professionals dealing with pregnant women were trained in emergency obstetric care. The impact was assessed using the CEMD of the 12 districts and the control group of the remaining 40 districts. It showed a 39.5% overall drop in mortality, mainly due to reduction in deaths due to complications of HIV infection, but also a 17.5% reduction in direct maternal deaths, mainly those due to obstetric haemorrhage and hypertensive disorders of pregnancy (Pattinson et al. 2019). This is a good illustration of the audit cycle and the part a CEMD plays in it.

Fawcus S, Pattinson RC, Moodley J et al. Maternal deaths from bleeding associated with caesarean delivery: a national emergency (a review). SAMJ: South African Medical Journal 2016 May;106(5):472–6.

Moodley J, Fawcus F, Pattinson R. Improvements in maternal mortality in South Africa. South African Medical Journal 2018 Mar 2;108(4):s4–s8.

Moodley J, Pattinson RC, Fawcus S, Schoon MG, Moran N, Shweni PM. The confidential enquiry into maternal deaths in South Africa: a case study. BJOG: An International Journal of Obstetrics & Gynaecology 2014;121 (s4):53–60.

Pattinson RC, Bergh AM, Ameh C et al. Reducing maternal deaths by skills-and-drills training in managing obstetric emergencies: a before-and-after observational study. South African Medical Journal 2019 Mar 29;109 (4):241–5.

Pattinson RC, Fawcus S, Gebhardt GS, Soma-Pillay P, Niit R, Moodley J. The impact of COVID-19 on use of maternal and reproductive health services and maternal and perinatal mortality. South African Health Review 2021: 106–19.

Dr Paily

Chatterjee A, Paily VP. Achieving Millennium Development Goals 4 and 5 in India. BJOG 2011;118Suppl 2:47–59.

Paily VP, Ambujam K, Rajasekharan V, Nair VR, Thomas B. Confidential review of maternal deaths in Kerala: a country case study. BJOG 2014;121Suppl 4:61–6. https://doi.org/10.1111/1471-0528.13000

Paily VP, Ambujam K, Thomas B et al., eds. Why Mothers Die: Kerala 2010–2020: observations and recommendations. Thrissur: Kerala Federation of Obstetrics and Gynaecology, 2021.

Paily VP, Ambujam K, Thomas B, Sekharan PK, Nair VR. Measures to reduce maternal mortality: Kerala experience. In press.

Professor Main

CMQCC Improving Health Care Response to Hypertensive Disorders of Pregnancy Toolkit, Version 2.0. www.cmqcc.org/resources-tool-kits/toolkits/HDP[6]

CMQCC Improving Health Care Response to Obstetric Hemorrhage Toolkit, Version 2.0. www.cmqcc.org/resources-tool-kits/toolkits/ob-hemorrhage-toolkit[5]

Main EK, Cape V, Abreo A et al. Reduction of severe maternal morbidity from hemorrhage using a state perinatal quality collaborative. Am J Obstet Gynecol. 2017;216(3):298.e1–298.e11.[9]

Main EK, Dhurjati R, Cape V et al. Improving maternal safety at scale with the mentor model of collaborative improvement. Jt Comm J Qual Patient Saf. 2018;44(5):250–9.[7]

Main EK, Goffman D, Scavone BM et al. National partnership for maternal safety: consensus bundle on obstetric hemorrhage. Obstet Gynecol. 2015;126(1):15562.[10]

Main EK, McCain CL, Morton CH, Holtby S, Lawton ES. Pregnancy-related mortality in California: causes, characteristics and improvement opportunities. Obstet Gynecol. 2015 Apr;125(4):938–47.[1]

Morton CH, Seacrist MJ, Van Otterloo LR, Main EK. Quality improvement opportunities identified through case review of pregnancy-related deaths from preeclampsia/eclampsia. J Obstet Gynecol Neonatal Nurs. 2019 48:275–87.[3]

Morton CH, Van Otterloo LR, Seacrist MJ, Main EK. Translating maternal mortality review into quality improvement opportunities in response to pregnancy-related deaths in California. J Obstet Gynecol Neonatal Nurs. 2019 48:252–62.[2]

Rosenstein MG, Chang S-C, Sakowski C et al. Hospital quality improvement interventions, statewide policy initiatives and rates of nulliparous term singleton vertex caesarean deliveries in California. JAMA 2021;325(16):1631–9.[8]

Seacrist MJ, Van Otterloo LR, Morton CH, Main EK. Quality improvement opportunities identified through case review of pregnancy-related deaths from obstetric hemorrhage. J Obstet Gynecol Neonatal Nurs. 2019 48:288–99.[4]

INDEX

Printed in the United States
by Baker & Taylor Publisher Services